I0796179

HEAL
WHAT
HURTS

About the Author

Maria Toso, SomaYoga Teacher through the International SomaYoga Institute, holds a degree in international communications from Copenhagen Business College. Born and raised in Denmark, she is grateful to call the United States her home. She lives and teaches in Saint Paul, Minnesota, where she raised her two children. Maria leads the Yoga Teacher Training program at Minneapolis College and runs a private coaching practice centered on her Heal What Hurts path—a somatic approach to emotional healing. Through group and individual coaching, workshops, and retreats, she helps others reconnect with the Divine Love within and transform long-held patterns of pain. To learn more about Maria and to share your experiences with the healing method in this book, please visit www.mariatoso.com.

HEAL WHAT HURTS

How to Heal Emotional Triggers

MARIA TOSO

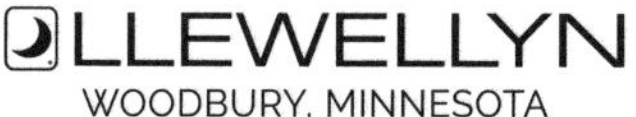
WOODBURY, MINNESOTA

Heal What Hurts: How to Heal Emotional Triggers Copyright © 2025 by Maria Toso. All rights reserved. No part of this book may be used or reproduced in any manner whatsoever, including internet usage, without written permission from Llewellyn Worldwide Ltd., except in the case of brief quotations embodied in critical articles and reviews. No part of this book may be used or reproduced in any manner for the purpose of training artificial intelligence technologies or systems.

First Edition
First Printing, 2025

Cover design by Shannon McKuhen
Cover illustration by Bella Toso

Llewellyn Publications is a registered trademark of Llewellyn Worldwide Ltd.

Library of Congress Cataloging-in-Publication Data (Pending)
ISBN: 978-0-7387-8149-5

Llewellyn Worldwide Ltd. does not participate in, endorse, or have any authority or responsibility concerning private business transactions between our authors and the public.

All mail addressed to the author is forwarded but the publisher cannot, unless specifically instructed by the author, give out an address or phone number.

Any internet references contained in this work are current at publication time, but the publisher cannot guarantee that a specific location will continue to be maintained. Please refer to the publisher's website for links to authors' websites and other sources.

Llewellyn Publications
A Division of Llewellyn Worldwide Ltd.
2143 Wooddale Drive
Woodbury, MN 55125-2989
www.llewellyn.com

Printed in the United States of America

GPSR Representation:
UPI-2M PLUS d.o.o., Medulićeva 20, 10000 Zagreb, Croatia
matt.parsons@upi2mbooks.hr

Disclaimer

The information and practices in this book are intended for personal development and educational purposes only. They are not a substitute for professional psychological, psychiatric, or medical advice, diagnosis, or treatment. If you are experiencing emotional distress, trauma, or a mental health condition, please seek the guidance of a qualified mental health professional or medical provider.

The author and publisher disclaim any liability for any harm, injury, or adverse effects that may result from the use or misuse of the information or practices in this book. By engaging with this material, you agree to take full responsibility for your well-being.

Dedication

This book is for you if you suspect that emotional triggers might be a culprit in your toughest relationship issues. May you be blessed with the courage and committed self-love necessary to go through the process of healing what hurts inside. May you feel the light of Divine Love always residing within and always there to be called upon for healing and releasing your old pain. So be it.

Contents

Exercises

Affirmation Prayers

INTRODUCTION

Writing this book has been one of the most challenging and rewarding experiences of my life. Typically when I sit down to write, the words flow effortlessly, as if they've been waiting for the right moment to spill onto the page. But writing this book has been different. The process of bringing this book into existence has been slow, deliberate, and deeply introspective as I continue to encounter more layers of old pain within. The subject matter—healing emotional triggers—is easily the most intense, difficult, and transformative journey of my life.

Healing emotional triggers brought me face-to-face with the rawest, most shame-covered places inside—places I didn't want anyone to see, including myself. And what I learned is this: Only the deepest loving presence—often far beyond my own—can reach and love the parts of us that feel most alone. My limited human self, operating from fear, shame, and separation, simply couldn't hold that level of pain alone. I had to call upon the Divine—not as a concept, but as a real presence—and in doing so I began to experience that I was also that presence. That Divine Love was not separate from me; it was in me, and it could move through me to heal the parts of me that did not yet know they belonged to love.

This work has drawn me into an intimate, living relationship with the Divine—not as an abstract idea, but as a steady, tangible force that is always with me, within me, and can be called upon at any time. It has been a journey out of separation and loneliness and into walking with God; a journey out of intellectual spirituality and into a love so vast, so all-encompassing, that if you asked me whether I would rather have been born trigger-free, I would say no. Because if holding each of my triggers in sacred, compassionate presence is the path to discovering the Divine Love inside me, I would choose it again and again.

Emotional triggers have been not only a central theme in my relationships but also a recurring challenge for so many people who have been drawn to my classes, courses, and coaching. This book is for you if you have also found yourself (over-)reacting in ways that feel beyond your control, particularly in relationships. Perhaps you've experienced moments where you feel downright hijacked by an emotional reaction that seems disproportionate to or rooted in something much deeper than the present situation—and yet you can't stop it. If this sounds familiar, you are not alone, and this book was written with you in mind.

This book won't just help you calm down when you're triggered. If you truly commit to this path, it will change your relationship with pain, with your past, and with your own inner world. You'll stop living on emotional autopilot. You'll begin to consciously create your life rather than compulsively repeat a sad storyline. You'll learn to meet your hurt with presence, interrupt old scripts, and become the author of a much more honest and liberated story—one that is true to who you really are.

As you apply these practices, something sacred will begin to unfold. You will grow more aligned with your true purpose—and with the Divine. You will become so lovingly present with yourself, first and foremost, that your presence with others will deepen effortlessly. You will feel that you are truly walking with God—as if the Divine lives inside you as a steady current of love that no one and nothing can take away.

You will stop grasping outside yourself for safety, for validation, for love itself—because you will know, not as a New Age concept but as a lived experience, that love is within you. As you bring gentle awareness to the parts of you that have not yet known love, you will slowly become more love, more light, and ultimately less burdened, less dense—freer and happier than you've been in a long time.

Recognizing Your Emotional Patterns

In my own life, my emotional triggers have surfaced most prominently in romantic relationships. But I have clients where emotional reactivity arises most intensely in friendships, at work, or with particular family members. I spent two marriages blaming my partners for my feelings of loneliness and abandonment. I lashed out, demanding they change so I wouldn't have to feel the unbearable contractions inside. Sometimes they would comply temporarily, but the relief was fleeting. Over time I began to notice a pattern: The same types of situations kept arising in an almost cyclical manner. It slowly, slowly became clear to me that the common denominator was me.

My saving grace was my very early involvement in meditation, yoga, and breathwork. I was nineteen years old when I learned to meditate at the Tibetan Buddhist Center in my native Copenhagen and twenty-one when a rebirthing breathwork session pushed to the surface painful, buried memories of two lengthy hospital stays that happened when I was four and five. It would still take me years to link that experience in the hospital when I was young to my meltdowns in my adult life, where my outer circumstances were sufficiently similar to activate that painful memory.

At twenty-seven I moved to the United States from Denmark after enthusiastically getting married after only six months of courtship. My then husband traveled a lot for his business, and it took some time for me to make my own friends and build a solid sense of community. When he forgot to call me before bedtime one night, I was transported back to that desperate feeling of a four-year-old being cast into outer darkness with no end in sight. Lashing out at him for this transgression—and soothing myself with vanilla ice cream—were the only ways I knew to help myself.

Looking back to that triggered moment, I know now it was a sacred opening. If I'd known then what I know now, I would have gone in and held myself in compassionate presence rather than lash out and numb out. I would have known how to offer the contracted knot in my solar plexus compassionate presence while calling on Divine Love to soften the contraction and release its long-held charge. But I didn't yet know what I know now about the importance of working directly with the emotional knots in the energy field of the body.

The process in this book is the tool I wish I'd had back in 1998. My hope is that it will also be the tool for you to bring compassion and understanding to the hurts that live inside of you. If your reaction to an emotional trigger falls into one of what I now call the three *outs*—lashing out, numbing out, and checking out—this book is for you.

You will quickly learn that while these *outs* are understandable reactions in the face of what feels like an absence of love and empathy, not only do they not heal your triggers but they also make the contracted energy you are trying to heal *worse*. Only love heals pain. This book will guide you back to aligning ever more fully with Divine Love and directing that love into the very pain you have been trying so hard to avoid.

The Three *Outs*

When we are caught in the grip of an emotional trigger, our default response, more often than not, falls into one of what I call the three *outs*: lashing out, numbing out, and checking out. These are reactive patterns designed to avoid pain rather than be with it, feel it, and thus heal it. We typically develop these behaviors early in life as survival mechanisms, shaped by traumatic experiences and the absence of the nurture and care we needed. When we resort to a particular behavior often enough, it creates what we in yoga call a *samskara*. A samskara is a pattern of behavior etched into the energy field of the body by repeated action—it's like an emotional groove we fall into automatically.

The first step in healing a samskara is to recognize it for what it is—to recognize that the *out* strategy we typically resort to is not who we are; it is a coping mechanism and can be healed. The path to healing both the habitual reaction and the underlying hurt is the same: loving presence fueled by our own inherent divine nature. You will learn how to do this in this book.

See if you can recognize your habitual *out*:

Lashing out: Do you ever react with a sudden, intense, and often aggressive or emotional outburst aimed at changing someone else's behavior? For those familiar with attachment theory, this is the reaction often associated with the anxious attachment style. People who *lash out* often feel that their sense of safety and security depends on external factors—in particular, a partner's reliability. In my case, why would I become so deeply distressed when my husband failed to call me before bed while he was out of town? My reaction wasn't just about the missed phone call; it was coming from the old unhealed wound of my childhood experience of abandonment. But due to my lack of awareness, I made him the source of my pain.

Numbing out: Do you ever use a substance when things get uncomfortable? Numbing out involves using external substances or behaviors to avoid feeling emotional pain. This could be through food (sugar is a favorite), alcohol, weed, nicotine, scrolling, drugs, or even work. The root of this response often lies in early experiences where our emotional needs were dismissed or replaced with temporary comforts. For instance, a crying child might be handed a lollipop instead of receiving the empathy they need, setting the stage for a lifelong tendency to soothe emotional discomfort with numbing agents. A loose definition of a numbing agent is any mind-altering substance you would have a hard time living without for thirty days. If, for example, you smoke weed or drink alcohol just once in a blue moon, it's probably not your numbing agent. But if you can scarcely go a week without it—and would genuinely struggle to go a full month—you may need to consider whether you're using it to hush important messages from your body.

Checking out: Do you head for the door or hide in your shell when things heat up? Checking out is a more extreme form of avoidance, where an individual disconnects entirely from their emotions and their body. This can manifest as dissociation or emotional detachment. People who check out are often described as having an avoidant attachment style. They've learned to protect themselves by withdrawing from painful feelings altogether, creating a barrier that prevents both connection and healing.

The Role of Shame

One of the most significant barriers to healing emotional triggers is shame. When we recognize that our reactions are disproportionate meltdowns or childlike, it's easy to fall into a spiral of shame. *Why can't I just handle this while staying cool and calm? Why do I keep reacting this way?* These questions, while understandable, often lead to stern self-judgment rather than self-compassion. Shame is a significant layer that we must address, and it must be addressed with compassion. You are not broken—you are learning to meet yourself with love instead of scorn or frustration. While we do have to get our *out* behavior under control, we must recognize the *out* as a way of avoiding pain—pain that is too much to bear because we don't yet know how to call upon Divine Love to cultivate the self-loving, compassionate presence that will soften the overwhelming contractions inside.

When we learn how to meet our triggers with presence, empathy, and love instead of judgment, we create the space necessary for healing. Shame makes us contract, hide, and definitely not want to address the triggered behavior. Presence and love make us relax, soften, and release the contracted energy. This book will teach you how to love yourself the way you were likely not loved as a kid, at least not all the times you needed it.

Emotional Triggers Are Trapped Energy in the Body

Emotional triggers are not an abstract concept; they are very real energetic knots that show up as undeniable somatic (felt sense) experience. They appear as blocked energy, often somewhere in the torso. Our life force energy (which in yoga we call *prana*) ideally flows effortlessly, like liquid light, through myriad channels in the body, intelligently healing and restoring any part of the energy field of the body that is injured. When we are emotionally wounded, we contract in an area of the body, making it harder for prana to flow freely there. In Ayurvedic medicine, it is said that every disease starts with a contraction or stagnation, a place in the body where the tissue is cut off from receiving sufficient prana. We find the same view of healing in Traditional Chinese Medicine, in which acupuncture needles are inserted into areas of the body where energy is not flowing freely.

When a traumatic or painful experience occurs, the body contracts in fear, and unless that contraction is consciously met and released, it can remain lodged in the energy system for decades or even lifetimes. I have seen clients in their eighties release reactive pain energy from experiences that happened when they were small children.

Contracted energy getting lodged in the energy field of the body happens in big and small ways all the time, and we must learn to address and release it on a daily basis lest it linger, creating both physical and emotional symptoms. Just as you would not hesitate to remove a splinter stuck in your foot, you must learn to address stuck contracted energy. It doesn't take much to accumulate contractions in the energy field of the body. For example, imagine being cut off in traffic. Your breath feels tight, your heart rate spikes, and your shoulders tense up. Once the immediate danger passes, you may think you've relaxed, but often a subtle tension remains. Over time these small, unresolved contractions accumulate, creating knots of frozen energy in the body. These knots contain information about the incident that you reacted to, like an energetic imprint of that moment in time. If left unaddressed, they not only perpetuate emotional reactivity but also eerily attract similar situations that reinforce the original wound.

What You Don't Heal You Will Relive

You will continue to attract versions of the same painful story until you soften and release the energetic contraction at its root. Whatever is present in your energy field—whether it's a memory, a belief, or an old wound—will shape your lived experience. If you've found yourself stuck in the same kind of dynamic over and over again, your body is not betraying you; it's revealing where love is still needed.

Triggers are not just emotional—they are energetic. They live as contracted knots in the energy field of the body, and unless we meet them with loving awareness, they will keep pulling into our lives the exact kinds of situations that confirm our pain.

An energy contraction is inherently uncomfortable and might lead you to "need" a drink when you get home or lash out in pain and irritation because your shoulders still hurt. Applying the process in this book will help you release contracted energy before it festers and creates emotional and physical problems.

The Intersection of Karma and Healing

These frozen knots of energy, or emotional triggers, are linked to the concept of karma. Karma is very much about the unresolved or unprocessed emotional energy that we carry within us. These energy knots act like magnets, pulling similar experiences into our lives until we address and release them. When you address a painful trigger that has shown up as a painful relationship, for example, you may find yourself losing your compulsive attachment to a person that fits the painful narrative contained in that trigger—or the person might start showing up differently. Working with our emotional triggers helps us take responsibility for what we are attracting and are attracted to. While this may sound daunting, it's also empowering. By bringing awareness and love to these contracted places, we can begin to dissolve them, much like an ice cube melting in the sun, and stop calling into our experiences the same painful scenario on repeat.

This view of karma explains in part why someone who was abused as a child may find their way into similarly abusive relationships as an adult. It's not because they deserve it; it's due to the compulsive repetition of a stuck energy pattern that keeps projecting itself out into the world as a very real-life experience. The healing of such an individual (and we all have our version of this) is under the hood. It's an inside job. We are not going to stop that loop from playing itself out until we shine light into the pattern and love into the wound. And that's what this book is here to help you do. The good news is that the Divine Love energy that is within each of us is infinitely more powerful than any blocked energy pattern, and as we commit ourselves to healing our emotional triggers, we gradually become more and more aligned with the Divine Love within and less and less likely to need an *out*.

Healing Requires Love

First and foremost, the healing of emotional triggers requires love. Big love. Consistent, dependable love. The quality of love that is at our core as a spiritual being in a mortal body. We must learn to combine present awareness, loving compassion, and alignment with the Divine essence within us, and offer it to the pain we experience. This process involves several key steps:

1. *Present awareness:* You can't do this work without becoming very aware of your breath and your body. You have to learn to notice the physical sensations in your body that are associated with an emotional trigger. This might be a tightening in the throat, a clenching in the chest, or a knot in the stomach. By becoming aware of these sensations, you can locate where the frozen energy resides and separate out from the wounded energy before it begins its downward spiral of *outs*.
2. *Loving compassion:* Once you've identified the felt sensation, the next step is to meet it with love and compassion. This means compassionately holding and sitting with the discomfort rather than avoiding it. Much like you would pick up a hurting child and

speak to them with the loving words you probably did not hear when you first sustained your emotional wounds, use words such as "I am here. I love you. I see you. I feel you. I've got you. I am not going anywhere."

3. *Divine alignment:* True, lasting healing requires more than just your personal attention; it requires tapping into the Divine Love within. By inviting this higher presence to surround and penetrate the areas of contraction, you begin to soften the knots and release the energy. In so doing, you establish a very real relationship with the Divine Love within—powerful, true love that doesn't judge, shame, or leave.
4. *Integration:* Over time, as the knots soften, lose their extreme emotional charge, and gradually dissolve in the light of your increased capacity for love, you become more aligned with your true self as a divine being in a physical body. This alignment reduces the likelihood of you acting out when triggered and enhances your ability to respond with love and grace. Less and less encumbered by contractions where prana cannot flow freely, the energy field of your body will become a healthier vessel for your Spirit to play in and you will enjoy more effortless manifestations of your wishes and dreams. As an absolute bonus, many other bodily symptoms may resolve. As prana flows increasingly freely and abundantly in your body, you will likely notice more energy, focus, and spontaneous healing of physical issues.

RACHEL'S STORY

My student Rachel felt embarrassed about a sizable ganglion cyst on her wrist that had persisted for twenty-eight years. She wore long-sleeve T-shirts in the summer to cover it up. As she moved through my program, she decided to try to love it every day. She spoke to it, saying, "I am here and I love you. You can stay or go. Either way, I love you." She did this for three weeks, then during a coffee date, her friend suddenly exclaimed, "Wow, your cyst is gone!" Indeed, Rachel hadn't even noticed. It was just gone. Loving compassion was the healer. We all have access to Divine Love, because it's who we are. It's what made us and what sustains us. We need only align ourselves with love and learn to direct that beam of compassionate love right into the most contracted, painful places in the body.

Beyond Reaction: A New Way of Being

As you heal, your capacity for self-love and self-compassion grows. You become less dependent on external sources for validation or safety, because as you soften and release the frozen knots that block your prana, your life force, you will find it much easier to cultivate a sense of grounded self-love within. This doesn't mean you will become invulnerable to hurt or disconnected from others, but rather that you will likely approach relationships from a place of wholeness rather than lack.

The more you align with the Divine Love within, the less you will feel the need to lash out, numb out, or check out. Instead, you will become a stronger vessel for love and compassion, both for yourself and for others. This shift not only transforms your inner world but also ripples outward, creating more harmonious relationships and contributing to the collective healing of the world. Whether or not your current triggering relationship(s) are appropriate will be revealed as you move through this process.

When a new client finds me and wants to work on their emotional triggers, they tend to want to know right away if a given relationship is worth fighting for. The best answer I can give is that you won't know until you begin to cultivate compassionate love toward your own pain. When your love toward yourself becomes steady and solid, there will likely be behaviors in others that just won't feel like a fit anymore. Sometimes that will result in others showing up differently, and sometimes the energetic bond will dissolve. Either way, you win, because you will be more closely aligned with love.

A Lifelong Journey

It's important to acknowledge that the Heal What Hurts path is not a quick fix or a one-time solution. Healing emotional triggers is an ongoing process, a way of living that requires a daily commitment to presence, self-awareness, and love. There will be setbacks, because shifting a habitual *out* is like filling in a deep, long-held groove while simultaneously carving out a new one. It requires steady, patient dedication, but each moment of awareness and compassion brings us closer to our true self, to the Divine within.

As you begin your journey and move through the pages of this book, I invite you to approach it with curiosity and gentleness. Whether you choose to work through the steps alone, with a partner, or as part of a group, know that you are not alone. This process is not just about healing your own wounds; it's about becoming the empowered, sovereign being that you truly are. From there you will effortlessly contribute to a world in which love, compassion, and connection are the foundations of our shared humanity.

The Journey of Coming Home to Yourself

The Heal What Hurts path in this book is laid out as eight steps. Therefore, I suggest you give yourself at least eight weeks to move through it. After that, you are invited to do all eight steps all the time, as needed. Each step includes a guided meditation. You can read the meditation slowly, but it will work best if you record yourself speaking it slowly and then playing it to yourself when you have the privacy to let it sink in.

The process of healing your emotional triggers is a gradual illumination of the energy field of your body and starts with something as simple as becoming more aware of your breathing and then adding increased awareness of your body. These two steps alone can bring up a lot more pain and buried emotion than you might expect. It is much like turning on the light in a basement that you haven't really taken a good look at in years.

You will notice things that you have pushed down (but that may well be the underlying cause of unexplained anxiety). There may in fact be times when you feel like you're getting worse, not better. It's sort of like how the middle stages of a big reorganizing project look much worse than when all the clutter was out of sight, stuffed away in closets, drawers, and boxes in the basement. It might be necessary and loving to put in place some therapeutic support as memories and unprocessed emotions surface.

The breath and body meditations presented in the chapters for steps one and two are likely to open you up to feeling more vulnerable, maybe even more volatile, at first. You may notice increased sensitivity to anything loud or crass, and you will likely need more peace and quiet, even more sleep. You will become painfully aware of what your primary *outs* are, and you may even feel like you are becoming more triggered initially. These are all normal symptoms of you arriving more fully into yourself, and for that to feel good, *self-love is essential.* You really cannot say to yourself too often some version of these words: "I love you. I am here. I see you. I've got you. I am not going anywhere."

It's easy to imagine that an abandoned orphan who has finally been picked up may need some time to trust that you are there with them and not leaving. In many ways, your wounds are like that orphan. By giving them your loving presence, you are establishing a sense of trust in yourself.

Journaling Prompts

Keeping a journal can be very helpful as you work through the Heal What Hurts path. Allow yourself to write down whatever you notice and feel. See what insights you uncover by addressing the following questions:

- What situations make you feel triggered?
- Do you *lash out* at the other person when triggered? Write down examples of when and how you might lash out.
- Do you *numb out* with a substance or with screens when triggered? How? Be specific.
- Do you simply *check out* and go cold when triggered?
- What is your default *out* when you are triggered?
- Be specific about how you *out* when you are triggered. The more details you can record, the more likely you are to wake up and realize that you are engaging in an *out*.
- Have you ever felt ashamed of how you reacted? What would it feel like to replace that shame with compassion?

THE EIGHT STEPS TO HEALING

The eight steps of the Heal What Hurts path are woven into the chapters ahead. You don't need to memorize the steps now—just let them land. As you move through the book, you'll find yourself returning to them again and again, until they become second nature.

1. *Breath Awareness:* Begin by anchoring in the breath. It calms the nervous system and opens a connection to divine presence.
2. *Body Awareness:* Scan the energy field of the body. Feel for areas of contraction, tension, or heat—this is where the pain lives.
3. *Skillful Coping:* Notice your habitual *outs*—the ways you lash out, numb out, or check out—and begin to interrupt those patterns.
4. *Locating the Trigger Knots in the Body:* Find the exact place in your body that contracts when you're triggered. This becomes your sacred entry point.

5. *Trigger Inquiry: Uncovering the Script:* Gently explore what story, belief, or memory is being reactivated. What does this place believe to be true?
6. *The Origin of the Trigger Story:* Ask how old the feeling is. Often a childhood memory will surface. Bring compassion to that version of you.
7. *Forgiveness:* Forgive not to excuse but to release. Let go of the energetic entanglements keeping the story alive in your energy field.
8. *Relationships as Vehicles for Growth:* Let your relationships become mirrors. Use what arises between you and others as fuel for inner presence and healing.

You will find these steps gently unfolding throughout the book—not in a rigid order, but in a rhythm that meets you where you are.

The energy field of your body is your precious vehicle for healing and awareness. The more present and aware you are in your body, the easier this work becomes. When I first started working with the energy field of my body, I had many blind spots—that is, areas of my body that I wasn't really able to sense and feel. Breathing practices, body scans, and Soma Yoga all continue to provide a pathway into a felt sensation of my body. Emotional triggers show up as disruptions—contractions in the energy field of the body. The contractions increase in intensity until lashing out, numbing out, or checking out seem like the only ways to discharge the pain. The goal is to catch the disruptions as early as possible. Becoming attuned to what is going on in your body is key.

Presence in the Body Is Paramount

You want to practice so much breath and body awareness that you become able to detect the triggered energy when it's subtle and you still have a choice about what to do with it. The answer is always to go *in* with compassion and love, but in order to do that, you have to be ready at a moment's notice. Anything that dulls your awareness of the energy in your body will only increase the likelihood that a trigger will flood you.

Alcohol and tobacco are probably the two most common remedies that Western humans reach for to avoid going into a state of feeling too much, but scrolling, sugar, weed, gaming, and shopping are numbing agents too. If you do not establish a practice of noticing any disruption to your energy flow, chances are triggers will overwhelm you. That is what the first two steps of the Heal What Hurts process focus on: becoming profoundly present in your body. Gradually this will become a new way of life.

When you become more proficient at detecting a trigger *before* it leads you to lash out, numb out, or check out, you will gradually establish a new habit of how you cope with a trigger. You will learn to take the *space* you need to be with yourself and compassionately speak to yourself with loving words as you allow yourself to feel the uncomfortable contracted energy just the way it shows up. You will learn to locate very precisely where in the body the energy is most contracted, and as you speak to this painful knot of energy, it will become increasingly clear what stories or beliefs you are holding onto. You will start to see in a very real way how these stories and beliefs have become your lived experience. Only as you clear these beliefs by calling on Divine Love and holding the contracted energy with warm and loving presence can you instill a new script, a positive affirmation that can truly take root only when it's not being crowded out by the negative stories that are contained in the old trigger knots.

The Freedom of Forgiving

This process opens the possibility of forgiving the humans you have gotten entangled with through the power of your trigger stories and likely also theirs. When we release resentment and grudges from our energy field, we can see more clearly what makes sense going forward. Are we in a coevolving dynamic with someone or are we perpetually driving the triggered energy deeper into our body? It might take a certain level of healing and increased awareness to see more clearly if a relationship is a manifestation of a painful belief or a sacred mirror that serves both parties in their evolution. While I have divided breath awareness and body awareness into two separate steps on the Heal What Hurts path, they really both apply all the time. If you have already done work with your body, you might be ready to work with both right away. If being aware of your breath and present in your body is new and foreign to you, then take your time with these two steps.

Step One
BREATH AWARENESS

We are born into this world on an inhale, an *in*spiration, and we will leave on our final exhale, *ex*piration. Our breath animates our physical incarnation for the duration of our physical existence—and the breath remains our connection to our divine nature, who we are beyond the material world. We can find countless stories of people who have had near-death experiences, including those who literally flat-lined and were considered dead, and they all speak of the "other side"—the state of consciousness from which we come and to which we return after experiencing being "in a body."

In step one on the Heal What Hurts path, we will practice breath awareness, which is another way of saying that we will practice remembering that we are spiritual beings and are always connected to the Divine. The breath is the most immediate way to return to presence. It's always available. And it's the first place we lose connection when we're triggered. Through our breath awareness, we can bring healing divine presence to anything that has contracted into a knot of hurt within.

You will learn specific pranayama (breathing) exercises and do a daily breath meditation. But even more importantly, you will simply notice, right now and as you move through your days, how your breath feels—inside your nose, in your chest, in your belly. Pay special attention to what makes your breathing rate change, as a change in breath (not caused by physical exertion) is often the first clue that you are triggered. Consider the possibility that you *are* the breath—the Spirit that is breathing life, light, and love into your earthly vessel in every moment. Visualize your breath as light illuminating your body, all the while sensing and feeling that the energy field of your body is an intricate manifestation of the content of your consciousness. In yoga, *citta* refers to the field of consciousness that holds your thoughts, emotions, and memories—often described as the heart-mind. Within the energy field of your body is lodged every unprocessed emotion. These energy knots are the source of your emotional reactivity, and we are here to melt them away with love, one by one, however long it takes.

Yawning is one of the ways we release stuck emotional energy. As you learn to work with your triggered energy, you will likely find yourself yawning more often and feeling release as you do. If a yawn feels stuck, you might visualize breath entering you as an incoming spiral. You might even trace a spiral with your finger on your thigh to help the breath enter the body more deeply and completely.

When You Breathe, You Spiritualize Your Body

This first step will guide you to a greater degree of awareness of your breath. In yoga, your breath equals your Spirit. In my native tongue, Danish, the word for breathing is the same as for Spirit: *ånde*. When you inhale, you bring Spirit in. As a newborn you took your first independent breath in, and when you leave you will exhale and release the Spirit from your body. We notice the same in the Latin languages and even in English. To be *inspired* is to receive an idea, to conceive of something new, creative, and fresh from the spirit world. To *expire* means Spirit is leaving, exiting. An expired gallon of milk means that life force (prana) is waning and is no longer as powerfully present, and at some point too much prana has dissipated and the milk starts to spoil. The practice we are embarking on here is one of becoming present, inspired, and full of prana, or life force, in the energy field of the body. We will use breath awareness to help us get there.

What If You Are the Breath, Breathing the Body?

In yoga we focus so much on our breath because the breath is our conscious connection to our Divine Self. We are all mostly so deeply steeped in the illusion that we are separate from Spirit that we see the breath as something we do to keep our physical form alive rather than who we *are*, the infinite essence of us that is giving life to this temporary, finite human form.

Contemplating the breath as who we are is a bit of a paradigm shift. You might say, "I thought I was this person, this age, this gender, this nationality," and you are, from a worldly perspective. Yet from a spiritual perspective you might say, "I have this vessel or instrument through which to experience and learn in this earthly incarnation, and I am currently breathing life, love, and light into this form so that I may participate in bringing Spirit light into the earthly plane. I, as Spirit, am here to help this particular human heal through loving presence."

Your Triggers Reside Like Frozen Emotional Knots in the Energy Field of Your Body

Your experience as the human body, the vessel, is of course very real. There you are, with a particular physical body. But the first step on the path to healing your emotional triggers is to realize that what is animating and giving life to your present earthly experience is Spirit, or breath. If you stop breathing, this vessel you currently reside in will soon turn to dust, just as milk spoils when the prana dissipates. The solid form of you is made of earthly materials that came together so beautifully when you animated it with your Spirit, and your body will come apart when you no longer animate it. When your breath leaves for the last time, you will expire and the body will die. You are formless.

When We Contract, We Block Energy

From the yogic perspective, you have been incarnated so many times and had so many earthly lives with a myriad of experiences that you have accumulated a lot of experiences and not all of them got processed or digested. Some action happened to you or was done by you, and the corresponding emotion (energy in motion) was simply too intense to flow through you and out. Instead, you contracted in self-protection and the energy got stuck as a knot in the energy field of the body.

This stuck energy is why we get caught in a loop of repeated experiences. Until the contraction is released by being bathed in loving, compassionate presence and the charge is gradually lessened, the painful event that caused the loop to be set in motion in the first place will play itself out repeatedly. In my experience, everyone carries around a substantial number of contracted energy knots that show up as patterns on repeat. Patterns are hard to break, but Divine Love within is greater than any negative habit and will be your best friend in this process.

You Are Not Your Reactivity Patterns

On the Heal What Hurts path, we are focusing on the contracted energy knots in the energy field of the body that have kept us in internal bondage. By becoming fully present in your body and aligning yourself with the Divine within, you will gradually separate out from the reactivity patterns that you carry around. You will witness them rather than being flooded by them. From the vantage point of being one with your Spirit Self, you can enter in and hold the parts of you that are not yet imbued fully with divine presence. Just like a loving parent picking up and embracing an ailing, scared child, if you show yourself love and compassion, your scared inner child will eventually relax in the arms of love: *I love you. I am here. I am not going anywhere.*

Divine Presence Melts the Frozen Energy Knots

You are essentially beginning an alchemical process of bringing your divine presence to the contracted parts of you that don't yet feel the full force of the Divine. You are transforming the leaden weight of your triggers into Go(l)d and melting frozen life force in the warmth of loving presence. By bringing your Divine Self deep into the dark corners of the energy field of the body, you can begin to transform the scripts running within each trigger. The meditations that accompany each step in this process are the way. This is a practice that you *do*, not something you read about and understand with your mind.

You cannot do this work from the level of intellectual understanding. This book won't help you unless you *do* the practices it offers. The process is a gradual shift out of the intellect and into a holy realigning of yourself inwardly with your Spirit Self, with your breath. The Spirit Self—the true self—is the silent Witness. From that perspective, you can approach those places within that are hurting, that are contracted, where life is not flowing freely through. Those are the places that constitute your emotional triggers, and they manifest outwardly as repeated patterns of conflict and painful dynamics with other human beings. Much of the time you are in a futile fight to get your unmet childhood needs met by someone else, and that someone else is very often an equally wounded individual who couldn't fulfill the role of a present and compassionate parent to you even if they wanted to.

To make the shift from overidentifying with your intellect to gradually becoming aligned with the Divine Witness within, you need breath awareness. When you become aware of your breathing, you will start noticing the state of being emotionally triggered much sooner, and you can then create space between stimulus and reaction. First you will learn to contain the urge to *lash out, numb out, or check out,* and over time you will learn to heal what is being triggered.

To begin this process, I invite you to become very familiar with how you breathe and consider how you can breathe more deeply and slowly and how you can use your breath to enter your body more deeply so that the energy field of your body can become fully illuminated and aware. Your goal is to become deeply in touch with what is truly going on within. Your breath is your guide to your inner landscape. It will be your guide as you learn to locate, release, and heal your emotional triggers at the root level.

Your Breath Will Alert You to an Impending Trigger

Most people notice their own breath only when they are winded or sick or feel nervous. I am asking you to gradually become more aware of your breath more of the time. Ground yourself in an awareness of your breath many times a day. Pause, close your eyes, and notice a few breaths. The goal is for you to have a slow, calm breathing pattern most of the time. When slow, calm breathing becomes the norm in your body, having your breathing pattern change will feel disruptive. You will immediately know that something is up, and you will be less likely to get tripped up by your emotional triggers because you'll catch the early warning signs that a trigger has been activated.

Breath Awareness Calms the Mind Chatter

In addition to becoming more aware of your breathing as you move through your day, you will also notice that when you bring awareness to your breath, you simultaneously slow down the incessant chatter of the mind. If you are completely immersed in the fluctuations of the mind, you cannot recognize and catch a painful story that is about to play out. When you become quieter inside, you can more easily hear when the mind is cooking up a painful interpretation of what is happening around you. You will start to notice the familiar scripts that are activated when you are triggered.

Pause again for a moment. Close your eyes and notice your breath. Notice the cool stream of air inside your nose and the warmer exhalation breath. Feel it. Listen to it. Are you truly exhaling all the way? Try again. Notice how tension releases from the body when you exhale more completely.

As you become more aware of your breath, you will notice how you breathe in different situations. You will notice how your breath might become a little short or a little shallow in certain situations or around certain people. This recognition allows you to ask yourself what's happening. Become more present within. Catch any *out* before you drown out the inner voice.

A Fast Breathing Rate Is Often a Sign of Chronic Tension in the Body

What do we tell someone when they're really upset? *Calm down, friend. Take a breath.* We instinctively know that if someone is upset, we serve them well by helping them ground their breath and presence deep in the body. What do we see when someone has been traumatized over a period of time? Their breathing rate is very fast and quickly gets even faster.

What do we notice about someone who is deeply asleep? That's usually when their breathing rate goes way down, because the body is fully relaxed and the breath has more unencumbered access to the body.

Practice Unconditional Love

As you start working with your breath, you might run into resistance to deeper breathing that could be born out of contempt for your body. It's important to recognize it as such so that you can love that feeling back into wholeness. If you notice judgments of your body showing up, lay your hands on your body where you feel the tension and say the magic words: "I am here and I love you. I am here and I've got you—and there is nothing you must do to receive my unconditional love."

When we do the yogic practices in this step—such as breath awareness, body scans, and speaking loving words to the body—we *will* bump into all the reasons we couldn't bear to feel our body in the first place. Body judgment is a frequent obstacle to presence and self-love. Please speak love to your body immediately and frequently if you notice body judgment arise.

The Other Person Is Your Mirror

Breath awareness is an essential step on the path to greater self-love, because it will gradually show you all the parts of yourself that you do not feel are worthy of love. Much of what we long for in relationships is for the other person to love us fully and unconditionally in a way that we ourselves cannot or will not. We often resent a partner for not loving and accepting us fully when we don't love and accept ourselves fully. That will not work. A partner will often simply mirror back to us how we love—or fail to love—ourselves.

Learning to Give Yourself the Love You Deserve

The pieces of us that we have exiled and deemed to be undeserving of love become tense knots that will continue to attract confirmation that they are exactly that: undeserving of love. Turning this cycle around begins with us learning to love ourselves—genuinely and unconditionally. That means love that has no agenda other than to love. You don't love the abandoned parts of yourself so that they will stop acting up or go away; you love them because love is what heals and you deserve to be loved and to heal no matter how long it takes. The meditation for each step on the Heal What Hurts path is the *how*. When you use the guided meditations, all of this will begin to click.

I suggest that you practice the breathing exercises in this chapter daily for at least a week and start noticing your breath as you move through your day. If you bump into self-judgments, return to this simple mantra: *I am here and I love you. I am here and I've got you—and there is nothing you must do to receive my unconditional love.*

Notice what happens when you gradually bring more awareness to your breathing pattern. Write it down. You are making an unconscious act much more conscious. This step alone will shift your ability to stay present and not get lost in painful stories.

A STORY ABOUT BREATH

Many years ago in one of my first meditation training sessions, I demonstrated to a new group of students how to guide the breath into the belly by laying hands on the lower belly. Next, I guided the students to hold their side ribs and feel the expansion of the rib cage with each breath. My intention was to teach the students to breathe more fully using more of their lung capacity, feeling the cadence of their breath.

After the breathing session, however, a young woman raised her hand. "I am so embarrassed to share this," she said, "but when I put my hands on my body, all I feel is self-loathing because of my excess fat. I hate my fat so much and work so hard to get rid of it." Tears welled up in her eyes as she courageously spoke these words aloud, then another woman chimed in that she felt the same, and then another. Others nodded.

I knew instinctively that only self-love could heal that pain, and we repeated the session and added this mantra: *I am here. I love you. I've got you. I am sorry I ever expressed anything but love toward you. Please forgive me. I love you.*

We can send love, radiating through our hands, deep into the various parts of the body where we wish for breath, Spirit, presence, and awareness to enter. We lead the Divine into an area of our body by being with that area of the body, bringing our presence and awareness to it.

Exercise

DIAPHRAGMATIC BREATHING

Learning to breathe from your diaphragm (and not just reading about it) will set inner change in motion. This practice includes two methods of diaphragmatic breathing: belly breathing and straw breathing. Each method is designed to help you deepen presence and soften the nervous system.

Belly Breathing

Most people don't breathe all the way into the belly. Another way of saying this is that most people don't fully engage and then relax the diaphragm when breathing in and out. Belly breathing encourages you to engage in diaphragmatic breathing. For many people, that will lower the breathing rate, and the nervous system will relax along with it.

PART 1

1. Grab your phone or another timing device.
2. Become aware of your breathing rate. Don't change it or direct it. Just notice it. Notice your inhales and your exhales. Maybe you can hear your breath. Where in the body do you feel it?
3. Set your timing device to one minute and count how many breaths you take in that period. (One breath is an inhale *and* an exhale.)

4. How many breaths did you take in one minute? Write that number down so you can remember it. This is your *initial breathing rate.*

PART 2

1. Keep your timing device nearby. Lie on your belly on a mat or rug. (Your bed will be too soft.) Stack your arms in front of you, much like you would to lie down on a beach towel, allowing the sun to warm your back.
2. Bring your awareness to the lower belly, below the belly button. Allow your inhales to fill the lower belly. Relax very deeply on the exhales. Feel your lower belly expanding like a balloon on the inhale and relaxing deeply on the exhale. If I were observing you from above, I would detect that your lower back is rising and falling with the breath.
3. Now set your timer for one minute and count your breaths again.
4. Did you take the same number of breaths as your initial breathing rate? Did your breathing rate go down? Write it down.

Straw Breathing

Here is another way of teaching the body to engage the diaphragm while breathing. The classic way of teaching this breathing technique is to use a straw, but you don't need one. You can simply purse your lips around an imaginary straw.

1. Sit comfortably with your back straight and your face, neck, and shoulders relaxed.
2. Inhale fully through your nose all the way into your belly, then purse your lips and exhale fully and slowly through the straw (real or imaginary). Don't force the exhale.
3. Holding a straw (real or imaginary) in your mouth, inhale slowly and fully and exhale gently through the straw.
4. Fill your lower abdomen as you inhale. Relax as you exhale.
5. Do this for up to five minutes at a time or longer if you wish.
6. Did you take the same number of breaths as your initial breathing rate? Did your breathing rate go down? Write it down.

Now, you might be wondering if you are breathing "right." I encourage you not to judge your breath, but simply to connect to it and gradually deepen it and slow it down. You will bump into areas of tension that prevent the breath from entering freely and fully. Just try your best to relax those areas.

During my years of working with often very traumatized women in recovery centers, I noticed that nearly everyone there had a very fast resting breathing rate. If the belly is tight with anxiety and fear, the breath has difficulty getting in, and we end up with a shallow, fast breathing rate. While every person is a little different, I have noticed that yogis who have worked with the breath tend to take around five to eight breaths per minute, while students with very stressful lives and unresolved trauma take as many as twenty or more breaths per minute when resting.

Do your best not to judge your breathing as good or bad. Just be aware of it. Awareness of your breath alone will shift your habits. Do belly breathing or straw breathing for five minutes once or twice a day.

Exercise

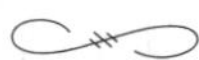

ALTERNATE NOSTRIL BREATHING (NADI SHODHANA)

Now that you have become aware of what it feels like to breathe more deeply into the belly, continue to breathe this way as you try this alternate nostril breathing exercise.

1. Sit upright on the floor or in a chair.
2. Find an erect spine by grounding into your seat and lifting up through the top of your head.
3. Continue to invite your breath into the lower belly. Recall what it felt like to breathe on the floor, with your lower belly expanding like a balloon on the inhale and relaxing deep inside with the exhale.
4. Using your right hand, lower the index and middle fingers to the palm. You will alternate your breathing between your two nostrils. As you inhale deeply through the right nostril, block the left nostril with the inside of your right ring finger. As you exhale, block the right nostril with your right thumb and exhale through the left nostril.
5. Now inhale deeply through your left nostril as you keep your right nostril covered with your right thumb, then cover your left nostril again with the inside of your right ring finger and breathe out through your right nostril.

6. Continue this pattern for several minutes. Take a short break if you get winded or feel uncomfortable, and then continue.
7. Guide your breath deep into your body and exhale all the way.

Do this exercise for five minutes once or twice a day. Sit quietly and notice the effect of your alternate nostril breathing.

Exercise

BREATH MEDITATION: BREATHE YOURSELF HOME

I suggest that you record yourself speaking this meditation slowly. That will allow you to focus on sensations rather than reading.

Allow yourself to become very still inside as you draw your awareness to the simple act of breathing. Don't change anything about your breath; simply notice how you breathe.

What does it feel like inside your nose as you draw breath in? Is there a scent around you? What's the temperature? Do you feel the breath more in one nostril than in the other?

Notice the sensation of the breath in the back of the throat. If it's still enough around you, can you tune into the sound of your breath in your inner ear? What is the sound of the inhale? What is the sound of the exhale?

Do you feel the exhale breath on your upper lip? Is your exhalation breath warmer than the inhale?

What is the subtle movement in the body when you breathe? Where is the breath most noticeable in your body? Do you feel the breath in your chest? Is your chest expanding and receiving the breath? What about your belly?

Draw your awareness to the belly below the belly button. Might the belly relax and soften to receive more breath? Is your breath slowing down a bit?

Tune into your rib cage. Can you feel the rib cage expand in all directions with your breath? Are you allowing the exhale to complete itself? Can you allow the exhaled breath to continue a little bit longer?

Feel your breath inside your nose. Hear your breath inside your ears. Feel the breath throughout your torso. Let all parts of your torso receive breath: the back, the front, the right side, and the left side. Your whole torso expands in all directions with the inhale and releases and relaxes with the exhale.

Notice how your mind has quieted down a bit as your focus has shifted to the breath. The breath has helped you become present. The breath has freed you a little bit from the mind, which always draws you out of the moment and into the future, into the past, and swirls around issues in your life.

Notice the breath, the invitation to become still and simply be. Notice how your body is gradually relaxing as your mind quiets down and the body is receiving more breath, receiving more Spirit. The healing vibration of your Spirit is now entering your body more fully.

Feel the cadence, the beautiful rhythm, of your breath in your body—from the moment the breath enters the nose to the sensation in the back of the throat, the expansion of the torso in all directions, and the softening in mind and body when you exhale. Can you hold awareness inside the nose, inside the ears, and in the body all at the same time? Can you feel all the ways in which the breath is showing up in the body, the gradual quieting down of the mind?

Now as the body softens and responds to the breath, it's more expandable and you can draw more breath in. You can fill up and feel the relief, the release, and the softening with the exhale. Find the true bottom of the exhale, where all tension leaves the body.

By inviting the breath into the body, the body is free to soak up the breath, the life-giving breath. With every deep inhale, the body is illuminated and revitalized. With every exhale, the body lets go of fear and tension.

Allow the body to receive more breath and release the tension it has been holding. Notice how the mind has quieted down. You are training your awareness to simply be with the breath, and you are training your mind to become still—or at least a little quieter.

Can you still feel breath in your nose? Can you allow the belly to relax completely so there's room for breath in the lowest part of the belly?

Do you notice layer upon layer of tension evaporating from the energy field of the body with the exhale? Over and over, you draw your awareness to the breath, the cool sensation of the breath inside the nose, the subtle sound of the breath inside the ears, and the rhythmic expansion and relaxation of the whole body as you breathe.

The body surrenders fear and anxiety to the exhaled breath. The body becomes softer and more relaxed with every breath. The eyes and the forehead soften as the mind becomes quiet and focuses only on the rhythm of your breath in this moment. All your awareness is on the breath. Breathe. Spirit entering and Spirit releasing. Beautiful, powerful, life-giving breath illuminates the body and heals the body.

Feel the breath inside your nose, feel the rhythm of the breath in your body, and notice how the mind has quieted down now that you have redirected your awareness from the intellect to the breath. Notice your capacity to redirect your awareness from the intellect to your breath, and notice how the mind relaxes into the breath.

Affirmation Prayer for Breath Awareness

Divine Love,

Please assist me in knowing you, my true Spirit, my breath, my life, as who I truly am.

As I practice breath awareness, I want to know myself, know you, within me, as me.

Help me today and always stay grounded in the moment with my breath,

Drawing life in, loving life, celebrating life, and exhaling all tension and fear as I surrender into your arms of deep present love in every moment.

So be it and so it is.

Exercise

BREATHE, RELEASE IT ALL

After years of working with yogic breathing practices as an integral part of my own (ongoing) Heal What Hurts path, I began to integrate a breathwork practice I call Breathe, Release It All into my daily healing practice. I first encountered breathwork in the early 1990s in Copenhagen in a series of one-on-one sessions with a rebirthing practitioner, so I knew how deep the practice could go. However, until 2020 I had not integrated Breathe, Release It All breathwork in a way that worked as a daily practice. I highly recommend giving this method a try, along with the previous breathing exercises.

While Breathe, Release It All breathwork is intense and, as such, is not for everyone, many of my clients and students find this technique incredibly helpful for releasing emotional knots and opening up to their own divinity, which is always there in the present moment when we release all mental chatter. Whatever lies right below the surface will likely be pushed up into your conscious awareness by the breathwork, so tears are not uncommon. You can modify the intensity of the breathwork simply by breathing for a shorter time or taking more breaks.

Breathe, Release It All is a transformational breathwork sequence that incorporates rounds of rhythmic breathing with intentional breath holds. It quiets mental chatter, softens stored tension, awakens the energy body, and brings deep somatic awareness to the places that most need your attention.

This practice tends to take you into deeper emotional and energetic layers more quickly. It often surfaces the precise areas in the body where contraction, pain, or unprocessed emotion has been held—making it easier to meet those places with breath, love, and healing presence.

While not required to move through the Heal What Hurts path, Breathe, Release It All breathwork can be a powerful ally for anyone who wants to deepen and accelerate their healing. It supports the release of long-held emotional patterns and helps amplify the body's readiness to feel, release, and transform.

You can experience this practice with a recorded version (available on my website and on YouTube under my name, Maria Toso) or in a group setting. We also incorporate this type of breathing in my Heal What Hurts seminars and retreats, where it supports the deeper layers of emotional release and embodied healing.

Exercise

BREATH REFLECTION

What was your initial reaction to becoming aware of your breath? Were you breathing faster or slower than expected?

Count your breaths again after completing the exercises and meditation in step one. Do you notice a change? Why or why not, do you think? Into which of the three *outs*—lashing out, numbing out, or checking out—do you most often fall?

Now that you've become more attentive to your breath, have you noticed situations in which it is accelerated? Slowed? Why do you think that is?

When in your day do you forget to breathe? What brings you back?

Step Two

BODY AWARENESS

Step two on the Heal What Hurts path will guide you into a deeper awareness of your body's energy field. As you dive deeper, continue to practice breath awareness every day and notice when your breathing rate starts to increase slightly in certain situations.

Pay attention to how your body feels when your breath is becoming constricted due to your body being in reaction. Now that you have familiarized yourself with your breathing rate and pattern, you will realize that the breath is the first warning sign that you're about to have an emotional reaction of some kind. If you can catch that early warning sign, you're much more likely to avoid the unconscious reactivity spurred on by the emotional trigger. This awareness provides you with an important moment where you can pause and consider whether becoming emotionally reactive is really how you want to respond. The more present you are in your body, the more choice you have. Triggers lose their reactive charge when they are met with loving presence.

Your Body Reacts to the Story Contained in the Trigger

In yoga we think of the body's energy field as a manifestation of our consciousness. Imagine that you are a person walking into a dark room in a part of the world where venomous snakes are known to enter people's houses. When you were little, you once got cornered by a snake and survived only because an adult walked in and wrangled away the snake. You realize that, lo and behold, it's happening again, because look: *Over there in the corner is a big, coiled-up snake.* The emotional knot of fear in your solar plexus from the near miss decades ago is reactivated, so even though you are no longer a six-year-old cornered by a cobra, the fear rising inside is very real and your whole body is in reaction. Any movement might agitate the snake. There is a very real risk that the snake will strike.

The shift in your physiology can be measured; your cortisol is rising and adrenaline is getting your body ready for a fight—or flight. You might feel constriction in your tummy, shallow breathing, sweating, and/or trembling. Then someone flicks on the light and the snake is revealed to be an old, coiled-up rope. You might laugh and say, "I can't believe I got this scared!" But your body really didn't know the difference between the coil of rope and the childhood experience of the threat of an actual snake contained in the trigger knot. The body reacts to the unresolved knot releasing its story.

So it is with all scripts that lie deep within trigger knots. When they are activated by an outer stimulus, we don't know the difference between what's actually happening and the body's physiological reaction. The script that has been activated is the one we respond to.

To heal the emotional triggers that lie within, you must become well acquainted with the energy field of your body so you can notice immediately what is going on within. The emotional flooding of a trigger can be delayed relative to how present and conscious you are. But once you are fully flooded by the physical symptoms of reactivity, it can be difficult to pull yourself out of the downward spiral.

We must create enough space between the outer stimulus and the inner response so that we can soften the degree to which we go into reaction, both inwardly and outwardly. We need time to go in and hold the contraction instead of having a knee-jerk reaction out of it. When we take some space from a situation, we can care for ourselves in ways that help the body calm down instead of becoming further agitated. Be aware that allowing for this buffer of space isn't the most natural instinct for you if your most typical response is to lash out.

Name the Location of the Trigger Knot

To heal our emotional triggers, we must enter the body more fully. The goal is that when someone says or does something that bothers you, you don't flare up inwardly or outwardly. Rather, you immediately detect your contracted reaction, that initial energetic response within the energy field of the body. You are with it. You can point to it. Is it in the belly? Solar plexus? Heart? Throat? You can place and name the sensation inside. Then you are no longer flooded by the feeling and can separate yourself from it ever so slightly, just enough that you stay connected to the breath and grounded in the body. Instead of detaching and checking out, you do the opposite, becoming more present and grounded in the body. This is particularly hard to do if you are under the influence of alcohol, so it's no wonder the most extreme cases of trigger drama often happen after imbibing. But even an excess of sugar or something as natural as an increase in stress or PMS can weaken your ability to stave off reactivity.

Learning to Name the Felt Sense

Learning to name the energy in the body is a new skill for many people and requires a deep sense of presence in the body. To acquire this skill, you must learn to more fully unite your awareness and presence self with your physical body. This is the true practice of yoga: deep, abiding presence inside yourself and staying with and in yourself, no matter what.

Yoga is not simply the practice of physical postures that can sometimes be done with the intention of subduing, disciplining, slimming, and strengthening the body. Yoga is to *love* and honor and be present in the body. Loving the body deeply and unconditionally is the most powerful healer. Staying aware inside the body is leading divinity into the body, into you.

Again, we must acknowledge the extent to which we place conditions on our love for the body. Many of us feel that we will not love our body until it is slimmer, stronger, curvier, or sexier—when it fits a particular culture's idea of what a body should look like to be desired and admired. The underlying hope is that this will lead to love and safety and protect us from the risk of being shunned into outer darkness.

Until we achieve some unachievable perfection, we are too often at war with our poor body. We may shame ourselves and feel embarrassed, looking for someone else to tell us that we are lovable because we don't truly love ourselves. Too many of us are unable to fully love and cherish our precious human body. Just as a child thrives in the presence of love, so does the body. We must learn to offer our body the same kindness and care—because love is the most powerful healer, and every part of us is worthy of that love.

Practice loving your body until you really do, and then practice some more. You are not just befriending your body; you are inviting the Divine to reside more fully within it. Your body becomes the temple where healing takes place. Love is presence. Deeply connect to your body as often as you can. Tell your body often, "I love you. I am here. I've got you. I am not going anywhere."

JIM'S STORY

In a private session with me, Jim balked at the invitation to love his body. "No way can I love my body until I lose twenty-five pounds. It's disgusting," he said. Jim was sixty-seven years old, and by his own account, he was carrying an extra twenty-five pounds that he had been trying to lose for years. At times he had succeeded through strict dieting and even stricter exercising, but eventually the extra twenty-five pounds always came back, much to his embarrassment and fueling his case against himself: *You are not lovable the way you are. If you are not perfect, you are not acceptable and not lovable, and I will be mad at you and embarrassed by you, and I will exercise you hard, you fat slob.*

This attitude carried over into Jim's relationships. Any sign of weakness or incompetence in those close to him really irked him, and he lashed out in irritation and frustration at the slightest infraction. Those closest to him often found themselves walking on eggshells.

"When I see fat people, I get so irritated. Slobs! Why can't they just quit stuffing their faces?" he would tell me. Yet when Jim was emotionally upset, he would reach for ice cream, and an entire pint was not uncommon. Often after visiting his dad, he would head straight for the freezer and plop down on the sofa with a pint and a spoon. He was using sugar to coat the emotional frustration he was feeling but not investigating.

Jim's breathing was affected by his contempt for his belly fat. His breathing rate was fast and shallow, using mostly the upper portion of the lungs. I asked him to place his hand on his lower belly and guide the breath into the lowest part of the belly, using the diaphragm to breathe deeper and slower. "When I place my hands on my belly, all I can feel is how much I hate my belly," he said. I suggested he talk to his belly like you would to a child who doesn't feel loved and safe: "I love you. I am here for you." He repeated the words with a mocking tone, so I took over and suggested that I speak for him, and he could simply keep his hands on his belly.

I said, "I love you, belly. I am here, and I love you. If you get much, much bigger, I will love you, and if you get much, much smaller, I will love you. There is nothing you can do to lose my love. I will love you no matter what. You don't have to earn my love by getting flat. You already have my love."

I asked Jim if he wanted to try.

Jim said quietly, "I love you, belly," then his chin quivered and he teared up.

"Do you want to try again?" I asked, and he did.

"I love you, belly," he said.

Then he sobbed and said, "I don't love myself. I can't love myself."

"It's okay," I said. "That's what we are learning here: to love ourselves unconditionally, to be with ourselves unconditionally. Nothing can heal without love. It's okay that we need to practice. Do you want to try again?"

He did. Quietly, he held his belly. Quietly, he wept for all the times his father's instructions had made him feel inadequate.

After the session, Jim seemed calm and grounded. The notion that he had to perform to a certain standard in order to receive love was an old belief that had played out repeatedly since early childhood.

Many of Us Were Taught That We Must Earn Love

Self-love is not easy. Unexamined triggers will always find a way to prove themselves. If we believe that we must look or act a certain way to receive love, chances are we will be drawn into situations or relationships that prove us right. If we are not in a state of self-love, we can easily confuse love with admiration, which is usually expressed as a compulsion to cultivate a persona that earns admiration from others, even though our wounded self is so longing to be held in love that doesn't require any performance.

Practice loving yourself, perceived imperfections and all. Make a habit of it. Remember that perpetual, targeted advertising is designed to invoke insecurity that will lead us to spend money on products designed to "fix" us in such a way that we will finally be deserving of love. Preying on human beings' need for love and acceptance is a billion-dollar industry that is growing by the minute. Why? Because no outer fix can fill the void formed when we do not love ourselves. Our only healer and guard against our wounded attempts to fit into a mold that we think can be loved is to become so present and self-loving that no one can persuade us that we need anything we truly don't. The work of healing our emotional triggers is a journey into our sweet, amazing body and into a deep, constant, consistent, ever-abiding presence. The body is the sacred road map for this work. The road map opens and shows us where we need more self-love.

Feel Your Whole Body as Often as You Can

The practice we will embark on this week is designed to make your body highly aware instead of numb and dull. You want to become so illuminated, so present in your body, that you sense and feel with great accuracy what is happening within. You fill yourself with your Spirit Light. You become more radiantly alive. You feel everything in more detail. To achieve this level of inner attunement, I invite you to contemplate the energy field of the body as often as you possibly can—not just during meditation or yoga practice but also when you take a walk, read a book, check your phone, or do the dishes. Feel your hands and feet, feel life itself buzzing like a low-grade current in your energy field all the time—all the time, even right now.

Stop for a moment. Be inside of yourself. Disperse your awareness evenly into the whole energy field of the body. Notice your breath. Notice how the mind slows down when you become present in the body and present to your breath. It really is that simple, but you have to practice quite often.

Everything in our modern world is designed to draw you out of the moment—out of your inner awareness—and into a sense of lack and desire. Our modern economy is based on you feeling empty and incomplete and consuming something outside of yourself in order to fill that void. If you allow this dynamic, you become a cog in the wheel of an unhealthy society that is destroying the planet with mindless production and consumption that has no endpoint. You filling yourself with loving, divine presence will lead to one less mindless consumer in the world. As you become increasingly present, you will lead the way for others. That sharing is where the healing of our world ultimately lies. Denying ourselves outer gratification without replacing it with loving, divine presence will lead to depression. Eventually we will break down and reward ourselves with something that will satisfy and still the incessant craving for a little while.

Please set aside time at least once a day to notice how your body becomes a little bit more aware and alert every time you pay attention to it. You become more aware of those little contracted energy knots in the body that you may have distanced yourself from because they feel so uncomfortable.

Become aware of which of the three *outs* you habitually turn to. Pay attention to the ways that you have drowned out your awareness of what is happening in the energy field of the body. Avoiding inner pain effectively means we are avoiding the feelings in the body. Gradually our bodies become dull and dense. The practice of contemplating the body is a way of gradually infusing it with loving presence—and this week's meditation will help you feel that more clearly.

The Body Is Always Noticing and Responding

Body contemplation is a turning point. From now on, you are going to start to listen and pay attention to the messages your body is offering. As the body becomes more transparent, more light makes its way into all these dense particles. You are consciously bringing your Spirit light, your deep, loving presence, into the body. This step in the process is all about bringing your awareness and presence to the body—over and over. You are essentially becoming a sacred alchemist who transforms the dense, contracted energy in your body into radiant love-filled energy.

Your capacity for presence and inner awareness will determine how well you can connect your body with Divine Love. It's a matter of practicing, repeatedly, as though you are patiently radiating a dense part of yourself with more light and gradually becoming more luminous. This union with the body is a crucial prerequisite for effectively healing and releasing emotional triggers. Be in the body. Feel into the body. Contemplate the body. Love the body.

I encourage you to practice the following Body Meditation several times a day. Learn the technique of body scanning to the point that you don't even need the guided meditation to shower your body with awareness. As with the Breath Meditation from step one, the Body Meditation will be most effective if you take the time to record it first, speaking slowly, so you can let yourself be guided by your own loving self. This meditation can be practiced resting on your back or seated with an erect spine.

Exercise

BODY MEDITATION: RECLAIM YOUR BODY AS SACRED GROUND

Welcome to your sacred body. Notice if some part of you is in resistance to calling your body sacred. Do you feel resistance to unconditional love for your body? Don't push that voice away, but don't let it take over either. Kindly tell that voice to please listen to your higher-self voice: *I love you, dear body. I am here and I love you so much. I am with you and I've got you, now and always.* Let this be your invitation to fully *embody* your body and really be present in your body so that you may be completely in touch with the sacred road map that your body is.

As always, start by noticing your breath. Notice how your breath enters your body and leaves your body in a rhythmic fashion. As you draw awareness to the breath, your mind starts to quiet down a bit. It feels good to be with the rhythm of the breath and relax the mind. Feel the breath inside your nose.

Notice the subtle sound of your breath. Invite your lower belly to soften and receive the breath. Notice any tension you carry in your belly, and gradually let it go now.

Let your awareness expand into the whole energy field of your body. Notice where the awareness easily goes and notice what part of the body is a little harder to be in touch with, to feel. Are you able to disperse your energy and awareness equally into the whole body?

Can you feel the energy in your hands? What about in your feet? Hold awareness now for a moment in your hands and feet together. Are the hands easier to feel than the feet?

Now see if you can feel your breath inside your nose while you notice your hands and feet in more detail. Feel into the tips of your fingers, still noticing the breath. Feel into the palms of your hands, still noticing the breath. Feel into the backs of the hands.

Notice your breath now and hold that awareness in your hands and bring awareness to the feet—into your heels, the soles of your feet, the tops of your feet, the tips of your toes.

Feel the energy present in your hands and your feet. Go deeper now and feel each finger in turn, all while noticing the breath.

Notice the subtle stream of air inside your nose, your hands vibrantly alive, the backs of your hands, the palms of your hands, your fingers, your fingertips.

Notice your breath now. Notice the rise and fall of your chest and belly now.

Notice your feet without losing awareness of your hands. Feel into your heels, the soles of your feet, the tops of your feet, and then the big toes, second toes, third toes, fourth toes, and pinkie toes.

Feel into the tips of all your toes, the tips of all your fingers, the rhythm of your breath. Feel into your hands and your feet, and now gradually draw this level of awareness from the hands into the wrists. Feel into your forearms and now your elbows. Feel into the elbows and forearms, the wrists and the hands, and keep this awareness while noticing again the feet, the ankles, the calf muscles, the shin bones, the knees, the lower legs, and the feet, and your forearms and your hands.

Notice the breath now. Bring awareness to the thighs and the upper arms. Feel into the inner thighs, the outer thighs, the hamstrings, and the quadriceps. Feel into the buttocks, the right buttock, the left buttock. Feel into your right hip and left hip. Feel into the pelvis, the lower belly, and the lower back.

Feel into the body from the waist down. Become fully aware of your body from the waist down. Now feel into the upper arms, the biceps, the triceps, the shoulders, and the armpits. Feel into the right shoulder blade, the right shoulder, the left shoulder blade, and the left shoulder. Feel into the right collarbone and the left collarbone. Feel your arms and your legs fully alive.

Feel your feet fully alive. Notice your breath, the stream of air inside the nose. Notice the belly button, relax the belly, and invite the breath deep into the belly.

Let the hard places in the belly soften now. Bring awareness to the belly button, the solar plexus above the belly button, and the stomach area. Bring awareness from the lower back to the mid-back. Bring awareness into the upper back. Notice the muscles around the right shoulder blade, the left shoulder blade, and the back of your neck. Bring awareness to the right side of the chest and the left side of the chest. Feel the breastbone, feel the right collarbone, and feel the left collarbone.

Feel the whole body from the neck down, vibrantly alive. Your hands and feet are alive, your lower legs and forearms are alive, and your upper arms and thighs are alive. You are vibrantly alive in your torso. Feel your body from the neck down, and feel the throat. Bring awareness to the chin and the jaw. Notice the lower lip and the upper lip.

Relax the tongue inside the mouth. Notice the lower teeth and gums and the upper teeth and gums. Notice your nose. Notice your right nostril, notice your left nostril, notice both nostrils, and notice your sinuses. Notice the right side of your face and the left side of your face. Notice your right eye and eyelid and your left eye and eyelid. Notice your eyelashes, notice your right eyebrow, notice your left eyebrow, notice the middle of both eyebrows, and notice your temples.

Feel into the space between the eyebrows. Feel into the whole forehead. Notice your right ear and your left ear. Notice the wrinkles and folds of the right ear and the wrinkles and folds of the left ear. Notice the scalp, the back of the head, the sides of your head, and the front of your head.

Notice the top of your head. Notice the whole energy field of the body together, from the tips of the toes to the tip of the nose, from the tips of the fingers to the earlobes to the top of the head. Feel your hands and feet, arms and legs. Feel your torso, back, front, and sides. Feel your neck, your throat, your jaw, your face, and your head.

Fill the whole energy field of your body with maximum awareness while noticing your breath. Keep noticing your breath. Keep feeling more deeply into the energy field of the body. Feel the vibrant energy of life throughout your body. Notice the breath bringing more and more life force into the body.

Notice every part of your body becoming fully alive and vibrantly imbued with Spirit awareness now. Bring even more awareness to the body, even more notice of any tense places that are blocking your awareness from entering. Gently find your way into the whole body. Be fully alive in every cell of the body now—from the soles of the feet to the top of the head and from the tips of the fingers to the tip of the nose. Everything is alive.

Feel your deep inhales and exhales. Disperse your awareness evenly into the whole energy field of the body now. You are vibrantly alive in the body. Soften the places that resist the breath, and soften the places that resist your awareness. Persistently illuminate your body with your awareness and notice the breath. Feel the luminous energy field of the body, everything in the body filled with beautiful life, everything in the body filled with life-giving breath.

Affirmation Prayer for Body Awareness

Divine Love!

Help me feel your loving light within every cell of my body, now and always.

I call upon your vibrant, luminous energy to fill my body and heal and release all areas of contraction and pain.

Assist me in showering my body with deep, abiding compassion so that every nook and cranny of my physical body may know you, radiate you, open up to you, and be you.

Spiritualize my body with your Spirit presence that my body may be a glorious instrument of your loving light and all density and darkness may be transformed into radiant light through your grace and love.

So be it and so it is.

Exercise

BODY REFLECTION

Think of a time when you were triggered. Bring yourself back to that moment. Can you identify where in the body that trigger lies?

____

____

In what ways have you numbed out so as not to feel your body?

____

____

What else might you do to bring more presence into your body? What practices might you incorporate into your life to do this? (Possibilities include long walks in nature, massages, warm baths, chiropractic care, acupuncture, essential oils, and vibrant food.)

____

____

Have you noticed a difference in the way you relate to your body after this week of doing the Body Meditation?

____

____

Which part of your body feels the most safe? Which part still feels guarded or hard to reach? What happens when you offer that part gentle attention?

____

____

Step Three
SKILLFUL COPING

In step three on the Heal What Hurts path, you will learn to stop before you reach for your *out*—your coping mechanism, whether it be checking out, lashing out, or numbing out—and bring divine compassion into the triggered state. You will learn to notice when you are abandoning yourself and begin giving yourself the loving presence you so deserve.

By now you have become much more acquainted with your breath and with the energy field of your body. You are probably noticing that life already feels a little different. You feel things more deeply and you notice things that you might have missed before. It can feel much like being a gentle, tender, open child in the world. That's a good thing, and it may mean that you are noticing an urge to stay away from harsh stimulation. Maybe violent movies don't feel good, or maybe loud or crass environments are too much for you. It might also be that the vibration of alcohol really doesn't feel good anymore or impacts you more than it used to.

Respect Your Need for Gentleness and More Stillness

What you are learning is to be so in touch with your own energy system that you naturally start to steer clear of the people, places, and spaces that are too harsh or too stimulating. You are getting to know a more open and sensitive version of yourself that emerges more and more as you shed the density that has accumulated over the years.

You are in the process of illuminating all numb corners within. With increased awareness of body and breath, you are ready to make a plan for skillful coping when you do get emotionally triggered, which will continue to happen until a given trigger has received so much of your loving presence that it loses its extreme charge and can no longer flood you.

In the past you may have coped by creating outer drama with the person who seemingly triggered you, numbing out, or shutting down. But with the skill of noticing and regulating your own breath and noticing your own body in a much more detailed way, you have the tools necessary for knowing earlier on in the triggering process that you're about to get pretty upset.

First of all, if you haven't yet determined what your primary *out* is, you'll want to get really clear on what your usual numbing behavior is. Typical ways of numbing out include intoxicants, sugar, excessive eating, porn, and shopping—anything to take the focus away from that awful triggered feeling in the body. What do *you* do when you are triggered? It will be obvious when you feel the first signs of a trigger rising: What would you much rather do than feel your body? That something you would much rather do is likely your primary *out*. I have been leading yoga teacher training programs since 2015, and early on a student confided that every time she sat down to do a prescribed meditation, her mind would scream, "Let's watch Netflix!" We all laughed because we all had our own way of avoiding being present inside, so we aptly named it our "Netflixing."

Watch for the Use of *Always* and *Never*

When you feel the early signs of being upset (the change in your breathing pattern and the energetic shift in the body), you can slow the whole trigger process down enough to become conscious of every step. You might think, *He said that, she didn't text me back, he hasn't called, she isn't there for me,* or the classic *You always…* or *You never…* When you use the words *always* and *never*, you are very likely in trigger territory.

If you feel yourself reacting to stories like these, that's when you want to pay very close attention and witness yourself. Do you suddenly crave a glass of wine, some weed, a cocktail, or some ice cream? Do you reach for your phone and scroll for the umpteenth time? That is when you want to backtrack for a moment. Ground yourself into your body, notice your breath, and ask yourself, "What happened? Why am I reaching for a numbing agent? What is it that I don't want to feel?"

Become crystal clear on what your *outs* are so they can't slip under the radar and distract you from receiving the very information you need to identify, heal, and release your trigger knots. Reaching for a numbing agent will provide temporary soothing, and sometimes that is what you are going to do—or even need to do. But be attentive. How have your numbing agents diminished your Light? How has your reactivity impacted your physiology and your relationships?

We are looking to stop the downward spiral, that predictable dynamic that leaves you feeling drained and ashamed. When you learn to stay present in your body, you can slow everything down enough that you can choose to feel and listen inwardly instead of lashing out or numbing out.

At this point, we are starting to fully realize that the outer cause of feeling emotionally triggered is the messenger pointing to a contracted energy knot inside that was put in place a long time ago and is screaming, yet again, to be held with loving presence in order to soften and release. If you are triggered and your body is already in reaction—you know the typical signs: shallow breathing, rapid heart rate, a knot in your solar plexus, tight chest or throat—now is not the time to start a discussion with the person who activated the samskara.

Stop, Breathe, Feel—Don't Numb Out

When you are triggered, tell yourself inwardly, "You are triggered, dear." Breathe. Stay as calm as you can. Feel your hands, your feet, then the whole body. Breathe. Lay a hand over the most contracted area in the energy field of your body and say the words we all long to hear: "I am here. I love you. I've got you. I am not going anywhere." A trigger knot has been activated and is now impacting your physiology significantly. Anything that comes out of your mouth (via phone, text, letter, etc.)

while you are triggered is likely not going to come from a place of higher wisdom. When the body is in contraction, the breath (and hence Spirit) is basically locked out of the house, and what you are left with is a scared child who is certain that danger is imminent, and your survival instincts start running the show.

If the body is in this triggered state, it is not the time to act, because any action you take while in this mode is very likely to be aimed at changing the behavior, thoughts, and feelings of that *other* person so they don't "make you" feel this way.

This strategy will not work. You know this. You have tried. It does not work.

Chances are you have also had a triggered person come at you with their demand that *you* be different so they can feel better. What is your response in this situation? That's right. It repels you. You want to back away, or you reluctantly find yourself trying to accommodate this other person to achieve peace fast—but chances are there is resentment mixed into the interaction, and resentment festers and breeds covert hostility.

When you first start doing this inner work of healing your emotional triggers, chances are you will not, at least initially, be able to calm down your physiology. Your breathing will feel constricted and a sense of anxiety or fear will wash over you.

When you feel these physiological changes, take a *huge* step back from the situation. If you are working with someone who is also doing this inner work, you might be able to name what is going on: "I am triggered. My tummy is hurting and I feel scared. I can't talk right now. I need to tend to this nervousness that is overwhelming me."

Over time, events such as these can become opportunities for coevolution and individual growth for you and the other person. But it's more likely that in the early phases of turning your attention inward and recognizing that healing emotional triggers is an inside job, you may want to create some space for yourself, some room to breathe.

Make a Plan for What to Do When You Are Triggered

When you are triggered, ideally you will choose to say to the other person something along the lines of, "I'm going to need a little space. I am not leaving you, but I need a little time to process what is going on inside of me right now." This may seem easy enough as you are reading about it right now, but in a real-life triggering situation, you may be convinced that telling the other person off is the dignified thing to do—or you may feel so shitty inside that you want the immediate relief you feel from your numbing agent of choice.

If you lose it, forgive yourself, but don't fool yourself and don't let yourself off the hook. This is not a one-off situation; this has happened before and will continue to repeat itself until you fully address the trigger in the energy field of your body. Be honest with yourself. Say, "I acted out, tried to convince the other person to change. It didn't work. It never does," or, "I numbed out," then name the way you numbed out. Say it out loud to yourself or to a good friend who is also doing this work. You can begin to take some of the power away from the numbing agent by calling it out. Name what you did, the immediate relief, and any negative side effects.

As you practice, you will become better and better at slowing yourself down enough that you are able to create the needed space. Your ego will likely try to convince you that choosing not to defend yourself or opting not to attack the other person is weak. If you do either, you will drive the trigger contraction deeper into the body and it will become even harder to disentangle yourself from its script.

Deescalating a conflict may be as simple as walking around the block, going to the bathroom, or sitting in your car. You *must* reconnect to your breath and your body to be grounded in your wisdom, your Higher Self. Without the connection to your Higher Self, you are an egomaniac on the loose, and your ego can cause a lot of damage very quickly.

I am inviting you to create a plan for what your skillful coping strategy will be when you are triggered. How will you create room to breathe? How will you stay grounded in your body and not fly off the handle or numb out? While triggers can show up anywhere and anytime, they tend to be activated by certain situations and people. Close your eyes and be real about your triggers. When and where do they typically happen? In that situation, what would be a way for you to create space to become grounded again?

Oddly, any intention to stay calm during a trigger storm, to step back and breathe, is often met with a more intense triggering situation. It can be almost as though the wounded part of you, or the *painbody*, is taking on the challenge: *Okay, bring it on. I will raise hell, and let's see if you can calm that down!* So don't be surprised if something happens between you and your favorite trigger mate that feels more intense than usual. Know that this is your moment to practice these life skills: the ability to disengage and take space, the ability to confront the wounded painbody's habitual way of getting attention, the ability to calm down, and the capacity to be fully present with yourself and for yourself.

Should you be in a relationship with someone who is also interested in doing this work, you might consider making a plan together to recognize when things are spiraling not just in yourself but in the other person as well. You might notice, for example, that when you and another person are in a trigger dynamic, you tend to fire off from the wound within and avoid looking directly at each other. Eye gazing reminds each human being of the oneness that exists behind the illusion of duality. The painbodies do not want to be reminded of that because it deflates the brewing storm before it can take hold.

If one or both of you can stay grounded enough, you might invite the other to stop and simply gaze into each other's eyes for at least one full minute. That will seem like a long time when you are in a heightened state, but it's really only sixty seconds. Do it. Be extra courageous and smile. It will be very hard for the other person not to return your smile. It may actually break the trigger spell that's taken hold and give you a moment to make some smarter decisions. This decision may still be to take time apart, even if just one person leaves the room, to allow your nervous systems to calm down.

However, this program does not require the participation of the person you are in a trigger dynamic with. You can do your own work and preserve your nervous system. You can break away and use the Skillful Coping Meditation below, which is designed to support you in the heat of the moment—when you are activated and need to calm your nervous system, create space, reconnect with your breath, and avoid reacting outwardly. I again recommend that you record the meditation first and have it ready to help when you are triggered.

Exercise

SKILLFUL COPING MEDITATION: SOOTHE THE TRIGGER WITH PRESENCE

Okay, (insert your own name here), I am here, I love you, and I know you're trying to cope with something right now. First of all, it is a *huge* step that you have been able to get yourself out of a situation that triggered you, hurt you, made you angry, made you sad, made you feel all kinds of uncomfortable feelings. Your body is probably in a physiological reaction. But you are here and I am with you, and you are not driving the trigger knot into deeper contraction. Bravo!

Now take a moment to simply notice your body. Name what is happening. How is your breath? How does your body feel? Where is the tension? Where is the fear? What is your go-to numbing agent when you feel triggered? Is it wine, sugar, your phone, or something else that helps you avoid the discomfort in your body?

Thank yourself sincerely for being able to extricate yourself from the situation. Now you are here and you are grounded enough to do this meditation instead of numbing out or lashing out.

Take a deep breath and put your hand on your belly or chest and really be present with yourself. Being emotionally triggered is easily as uncomfortable as physical pain, if not more so, and there's no doubt that the feeling of being triggered is the beginning of all addictions. No one wants to feel like a trembling child in an adult body. But know that I am holding you with my love now. I am with you and in you.

Let yourself notice what, if any, numbing agent is calling to you right now. What might you habitually reach for to make this feeling go away or at least soften a bit?

Remember that whatever this numbing agent is, it will be there waiting for you should you choose it. But notice that you have a choice, right now, to simply be. Breathe.

Your Divine Spirit Self, the real healer, is right here. Breathe. Your Divine Spirit Self is truly right here with you. You know how to connect to your Higher Self. You start by noticing your breath. Deepen and slow down your breath. Close your eyes and let your breath be all that is. Breathe. This too shall pass, but this painful feeling inside of you right now needs your attention, love, and presence. So simply be and breathe.

Bring your awareness to your lower belly now. Invite your breath into the lower belly. Relax your belly. Invite the breath in even deeper: deep breath in and deep, long breath out.

Being triggered is most often associated with a feeling of butterflies in the tummy or tightness in the chest and belly. Let your hands rest on your belly and feel the gentle rise and fall of the belly.

Slowly draw breath deeply in and then let out a long, deep exhale. It can even be an audible sigh. Do this several times. You are dissipating some of the contracted energy, softening the charge a little bit, so that it becomes more manageable.

Let's do it again: Inhale deeply through the nose and into the belly and breathe slowly all the way out through the mouth.

Allow your belly to be receptive, soften, and relax.

Feel your deep breath entering the body and exhale all the way. Already a little bit better. More grounded *in* you. More there *for* you. More there *with* you.

Keep letting your awareness be very present in the whole of the body.

Keep redirecting your attention from your racing mind to this moment.

If you find yourself reading the other person their rights or composing your defense or attack, then gently redirect your attention.

Say out loud: "It's not about (person's name). (Name) is neither good nor bad. It's about me."

Say out loud to yourself: "I am here. I love you. I am not leaving you." Feel yourself. Feel the pained, contracted place within. Talk to this place. Your samskara has been blown open. This is a holy moment. Breathe into this hurting part of yourself. Say again: "I am here. I love you. I am not leaving you."

Know that you have the mastery to simply be right here, to simply breathe. This nearly overwhelming feeling of agitation is temporary. This too shall pass. Slowly breathe through it right now. Become aware of your hands and your feet. Where are your arms and your legs? Notice where your belly is tight. Let it soften now so you can breathe deeper into the belly.

Remember this: When you're upset and triggered, you're fully identifying with the wounded part of yourself that needs your Divine Self, your deep love, for healing.

Separate a little from this place that is so hurt and wounded right now. Notice it and remember that your true nature is the one that's breathing you right now. Feel your breath. That is you.

Like a loving mother holding a crying baby, let the Spirit in you breathe a loving presence into you. Let the Spirit in you wrap loving Spirit arms around this wounded place within.

See if you can align yourself now with both pieces of yourself: this beautiful breathing self that is fully present and calm and this agitated, scared, upset, contracted part of you that has been activated by outer circumstances because it needs healing.

Simply say, over and over: "I am here for you. I love you and I am not going anywhere. I am here for you. I love you. I am not leaving you."

You can say it out loud or inwardly, whatever is appropriate for your situation.

"I am here. I am here. I know you're hurting. I know you are sad. I know you are angry and upset. I'm not leaving." Keep breathing deep into the belly now.

Allow yourself to feel this pained place within. Hold it in deep presence and love.

Your Higher Self is with you. You are upset, and understandably so, because there is a deep wound there, but it's not all of you. It's a part of you.

Breathe calmly and deeply. You are gradually realigning yourself with your Spirit Self.

Let your hands find the place in your body where the contraction or emotional tension feels most intense.

Notice the presence of spiritual energy in your hands.

Your hands radiate beautiful Light and Love directly into the places in your energy field that are in turmoil right now.

Remember that these places are showing themselves because they need love and presence. Only loving presence can heal you.

You are learning to love yourself deeply. This takes practice; please stick to it. Stay present with the pain. Envelop the pain in love. Even more. Hold. Feel it. Be with it.

Your hands are radiating Divine Love. Your breath is breathing love into the darkness and despair.

You are okay. All is well and this too shall pass.

Stay with it here.

Now be fully aware of your entire body. Feel your legs and your arms. Feel your hands and your feet. Feel the torso and feel the relatively smaller, defined part of you that is contracted, scared, and in reaction. This part of you isn't all of you.

It is a part of you and you do have the Spirit capacity to love this place and hold it now.

Keep feeling into it and be with it unconditionally.

It's okay to cry. It's okay to feel angry, sad, lonely, or scared.

You have come here to heal this place within you. This place needs to be wrapped in love, not shoved away, numbed out, or silenced. Be with this samskara. Hold it in your infinite loving-kindness.

Notice your breath gradually calming down now.

Look around you and name what you're seeing. Let your eyes wander from object to object. Name each object.

You are safe. At this moment you are safe. Keep going, look around. Name what you see. You can name it out loud or inwardly.

When you have made a 360-degree circle around you, naming all the things that are around you, feel your whole body again.

Feel what you're sitting on, or standing on, or lying upon.

Feel the earth's solid support. Feel where your body is touching the earth right now.

Bring your awareness to the part of your body that's touching something right now.

Feel that support. Feel the support in this moment while being fully aware of what's around you. You are gradually calming down. You're separating out a little bit from that most contracted place within. Let yourself soften inside.

Keep encouraging the breath all the way into the lower belly. Let the belly soften. Allow the mind to quiet down. It doesn't have to figure anything out right now, no planning right now.

You don't have to say anything, write anything, text anything, or do anything now.

Right now you are tending to a place in yourself that truly needs you.

Hold this place within with deep, patient love. Say to yourself, "I am here for you. I am not leaving you. I've got you. I'm here. I am not leaving. I love you."

Feel this deep love you are capable of that is *you* at the core. Keep breathing deeply. Feel the breath in the nose, hear the breath in your ears.

Invite breath in, bring it into the fullness of the belly, breathe into the belly, and give yourself time to exhale. As you exhale, let the tension evaporate from the body.

This is huge. You are learning to master something that has overwhelmed you many times before. Be here. Hold yourself in love.

And now, using your own name, with your hands on the part of your body that feels this turmoil, that feels the most contracted, say this mantra inwardly or out loud:

"I love you. I'm here. I am right here, I am right here. I am holding you and I'm staying with you. I am deeply connected to Divine Source. There's nowhere for you to fall because I've got you. I'm breathing with you. I am breathing you. You can relax into me. I've got your back."

Breathe all the way into the belly now. Sigh out loud on the exhale and let go of the tension now. Continue to feel the support of the earth below you. Disperse your awareness evenly throughout your body and listen to the rhythm of the breath of the world around you. Listen to the sounds around you.

Everything is okay. There's no need to respond to anything now. The only thing that matters now is calming your body.

Allow your breath to connect you to the Divine Love within you and all around you.

Your greatest pain *is* in the process of transforming through the power of loving presence. You are in transformation. Your samskaras are softening.

Now let yourself rest. Take an Epsom salt bath or go for a walk if you can.

Drink a tall glass of water, then another. Water helps clear tension and calm you. It's not yet time to engage with that other person.

Give it some space.

Exercise

SKILLFUL COPING REFLECTION

Now that you have become more aware of your breath and your body in various situations, can you name some signs that you're triggered? What happens to your breath? Where do you feel it in your body?

What numbing agents do you notice yourself reaching for when you become triggered? (This could be anything from sugar to tobacco to exercise to shopping.)

What is your plan to take space if you become triggered? Where can you go?

What can you say to the other person to take space in a calm, collected, and neutral way that doesn't invite drama?

Are you able to listen to your body and tune into the contracted knots in the energy field of your body? Can you communicate love verbally and energetically to the contractions?

Affirmation Prayer for Skillful Coping When Triggered

Divine Love!

I call upon your powerful presence within me as I feel my body and my breath.

I know you are here within me, soothing me and spreading your glorious, luminous light inside my tormented energy field.

I am triggered. I feel contracted in areas of my body, and I feel the old familiar feelings of hurt inside—the ones I want to run away from, the ones that scare me, make me lash out, numb out, check out.

I want to stay right here. With you. With God. With the glorious, loving light of presence within my heart.

I now allow the loving light in my heart to spread throughout my body.

Embrace my contracted energy and hold me deeply in loving presence.

I am full of your Light. I am full of your Love.

So be it and so it is.

A STORY ABOUT TRIGGERS

Rina, who worked as a nurse, shared a story with me about being asked for a new prescription for pain medication. Her patient claimed that he had lost his prescription, and she became very upset by his request. As we investigated why she had gotten so upset, she suddenly blurted out, "He was lying! He was clearly taking me for an idiot."

The charge was palpable; her words carried pain and tension. I asked her to pause, to feel that sentence, that story, in her body. I asked her to close her eyes and relax out of the narrative and feel into her body. I repeated what she had said: "He takes me for an idiot, he takes me for an idiot, he thinks I am an idiot." As I repeated this story and she experienced the feelings within her body, we further activated this old wound, or samskara. As she felt the energy activated in the body, she experienced sadness rather than anger.

"Is this the first time you have felt that someone took you for an idiot?" I asked.

She said, "No, when I feel this feeling in my body, I am reminded of feeling this way all the time as a kid: when my dad looked at me a certain way, the way my brothers talked to me, the youngest and only girl in the family." Rina's face tensed, then she cried. She released a bit of the painful programming from her past, the message "I am being taken for an idiot."

Once we recognize how our experiences and memories contribute to our interpretation of a present situation, it's possible to question the story. I said to Rina, "'He takes me for an idiot' is one possible way of viewing the conversation that took place. What are other ways to think about this patient who was requesting a new prescription for pain medication?"

Rina was much softer now and said, "He was in pain. He wanted his pain to stop. He wanted to feel better. Maybe he was lying; maybe he wasn't. I don't know. But I know that he wanted to stop the pain."

"Now what feelings arise when you think of it that way?" I asked.

"Compassion," Rina said. "The anger is gone, and I feel sad for him."

Two things were accomplished. Rina was able to feel the samskara within her that led her to expect that someone would lie and "take her for an idiot"—which means that the next time she interprets a situation in the same way, something in her will likely pause and think, "Hmm, is this my habitual way of interpreting a situation or is this person really taking me for an idiot?"

The other thing that happened was that Rina went from angry to compassionate, a much softer state of being. The emotion of anger is often accompanied by the release of stress hormones in the body, which can cause hypertension and also the urge to take the edge off that tense feeling with a glass of wine, shopping, or eating, for example. The feeling of compassion toward another is a much gentler vibration that often leads to compassion toward the self and others. The healing is underway.

Step Four

LOCATING THE TRIGGER KNOTS IN THE SACRED ROAD MAP OF THE BODY

You are gradually becoming more skilled and better equipped to move even deeper into the energy field of the body. Step four on the Heal What Hurts path will teach you to locate the samskaras in the energy field of your body. As you begin to trust the way your body is communicating with you, it becomes a sacred road map leading you to the places that need your divine presence to transform.

The energy field of your body is your sacred road map. Keeping your body healthy and nourished will enhance the signals you are receiving. Numbing the body with dense and dull foods, sugar, intoxicants, electronics, or a lack of daily movement will make it harder for you to get accurate information.

If you let it, the treasure map of your body will show you very precisely where the hidden scripts lay buried deep inside your samskaras. This requires you to be both curious and empathic. During this step, you will learn to locate the energetic location of a samskara, and when you do, it may reveal to you information about when and where the samskara script originated. Or if the samskara is preverbal, it may simply show up as an energy that needs presence to transform. Let it be an exploration driven by love.

Often a particular script is activated very easily within you. It may seem like a particular individual is triggering this script, but in most cases you will find that the script is older than your relationship with your current villain. If you are lucky enough to be doing this program with someone else, they may be able to reflect back to you the story that appears to be driving your emotional responses.

While you want to keep the focus on your own inner work, it can be interesting to look around and see how nearly everyone you know seems to have a certain story that they live out over and over.

When you realize that you are the common denominator in each recurring emotional pattern or trigger, it can be humbling. But this recognition is also the key to lasting change. It invites you to take responsibility on a whole new level and to begin turning inward—not only for the answers, but because the real healing work can only happen inside you. This is not to be done with shame and judgment, but with great love and empathy.

Samskaras open and show us their story when we surround and hold them with loving presence. When we meet them with exasperation, our own or someone else's, they contract and lock up tight from the inside to protect this wounded soul area from further injury. Only love heals, softens, opens, and releases. Shaming and judging contract and harden.

The (thankfully dying) patriarchal model of pitting kids against each other from an early age, teaching them the survival of the fittest and public ridicule of the weakest, has produced samskaras of epidemic proportions in humankind. We may all manage to look tough on the exterior, but that tough look doesn't come from inner strength. It's actually a tough exterior guarding deep soul injuries that react time and again. We are all desperately looking to get our unmet childhood needs met by other adults who also didn't have their childhood needs met.

Healing is possible only when we each learn to love and hold ourselves and our samskaras in unconditional love. Only when we have mastered the heavenly art of holding, healing, and releasing our own pain can we ever truly do that for others in an unconditional manner. If we treat our own samskaras as a matter of embarrassment to be hushed and pushed deep down, then we will give off that same vibe toward the pain of others and of Mother Earth herself.

Not feeling and healing our samskaras leads us to be less and less compassionate and caring and more and more self-righteous in our callous treatment of those who are wounded and weak, whether inside of ourselves or in the outer world.

The current state of the climate is a direct consequence of how we treat our own tenderness and our refusal to be honest about the impact of our actions. Everything from the survival of the planet to the survival of our relationships to ourselves and others hinges on our willingness to stop lashing out, numbing out, or checking out. We must become intimately familiar with the sacred road map of our bodies. We cannot afford to live in such a way that the body is not heard.

In my work with students and clients, I've observed a sharp rise in panic attacks and anxiety-related symptoms in recent years. Our bodies are screaming for attention. By this I mean that the whole energy field of the body-heart-mind urgently needs our conscious attention. We need to hone our observational skills by focusing our awareness on the energy field generated by our own body and noticing how every feeling, thought, and action reverberates within that field.

If you have come this far on the Heal What Hurts path, you have, perhaps inadvertently, decided to be part of the solution. This week we're going to go a little deeper into the energy field of the body by figuring out what is bound up in the story of a triggered moment and explore what might have been the first time we felt the samskara that has been acting up.

Making a samskara's acquaintance is an almost magical process. Your entry into a samskara that is asking for your healing presence is through the portal of one of your triggered moments. As you progress in your work with your emotional triggers, you will come to realize that the triggered moment is not merely a terrible incident to be survived; it's an invitation to bring your Divine Self deep into the places within you that don't yet know Spirit.

Take a moment to recall a recent triggering situation that holds a strong emotional charge for you.

In the Sacred Road Map Meditation later in this chapter, I will guide you through a contemplation of your energy field and help you identify the physical location of any lingering emotional charge. It will likely feel like a contraction in your energy field, a block where energy cannot flow freely.

The energy contraction of a samskara is not a comfortable feeling. In fact, it's the exact feeling we all try so very hard to avoid by lashing out, numbing out, or checking out—anything to lessen the charge. But what you will come to learn is that the only true medicine that will lessen the charge over time is your loving presence. And by your loving presence, I mean your Divine Self essence—the Witness, the observer, the breath within you that you have come to know so much better through the breathing exercises in step one, and your body that you are also so much more present in after doing the second step.

We often associate shame with our samskaras, so it's not a place you're naturally going to want to hang out in. But I'm asking you to be with it anyway. Because this is the place within you that is hurting and it truly needs your loving presence. It needs your Spirit energy to surround it with love and acceptance. The holding and reassurance that you are here to listen and not judge will allow your samskara to tell its story—a story that is likely to be from a very young age.

When you ask this place, "When have you felt this before?" you will probably be taken back to a young age when this feeling first appeared. It will be painful to recall your defenseless younger self that needed so very much to feel loved and safe and like you belonged. Know this: Anything less than feeling loved, safe, and like you belong is devastating. It was devastating to you when you were a child and it's devastating to you now. Humans can learn to tolerate, or more often medicate, the absence of these fundamental human qualities, but we simply cannot thrive if we do not feel safe, loved, and like we belong.

I have never seen a student move through this phase of healing emotional triggers without crying. So tears have to be okay. Pain has to be okay. Know that it's temporary. You are discovering something really important. You will come to understand the samskara script that has been triggered many times in your adult life.

This script lives inside this little contracted place within. It's an energy pattern, and you *will* experience compulsive repetition of this story until the samskara has been loved back into the wholeness of your spirit being. Your samskaras do not vanish on their own. They soften, relax, and release when showered with enough love.

This is the sacred work of spiritualizing yourself—bringing your loving, compassionate, Spirit-infused awareness to the painful places inside. That is the medicine: your loving presence. It softens, soothes, and slowly unwinds what has been held in contraction.

I will say it again: The only effective healer is your own loving, healing presence—not lashing out, not numbing out, and not checking out. You will want to do one of those three things until you stop and love yourself instead, with deep, loving, compassionate presence.

This place within, this contracted samskara, has been pushed down for a long time and you will need to hold it and hold it and hold it until it feels safe with you. Imagine the samskara is a neglected, lonely child finally being picked up from an orphanage. Give this child all the time needed to trust you, to relax into you, to know that you are not going anywhere. And know this: Until it is healed, your samskara will get activated again—and likely sooner rather than later.

Before a pattern breaks, it tends to contract and sometimes it seems like it's getting worse before it gets better. I would suggest that it's not really getting worse; you are just noticing it and taking full responsibility for it. You are less numbed out and more aware of when you feel the early signs of a trigger. You are also building your tolerance for being with the initial discomfort of an activated trigger. This is hard, and no one teaches us how to do this, so you are learning right now. Let yourself be a student of this process and trust that you really are on the road to healing your emotional triggers.

The danger zone is the moment between the activation of a trigger and the time it takes you to ground yourself enough to bring your full loving awareness into your body. Rule number one: Pay attention to your breath. When your breath is shallow, your higher awareness gets cut off, and insecurities and ingrained habits will likely take over.

You are learning a new skill here, and it will take a while to master it. The breath and body scan practices from steps one and two will be your best tools. If you can keep your breathing deep and slow and be deeply present in your body, you will be much less likely to act out of panic and fear.

This is not an overnight fix, and as I mentioned, you will still experience being triggered, but it's not going to blow up quite the same. When the trigger starts to act up, you may find that you are not as quick to condemn it or react to it.

You may be a little less likely to lash out at some perceived villain, and I promise you, the villain is not going to give this small, scared child what they need. You are. Begging the villain to be the loving presence that you won't be for yourself never works. It never works.

You are going to hold this sweet little vulnerable you that is contained within the samskara energy. This little person who was wounded and not taken care of properly at the time of injury did not have the skills to hold themselves. Now your divine presence self gets to come in and hold this scared child-like aspect of you.

This will make more sense as you move through the Sacred Road Map Meditation later in this chapter, where you will enter deep into the energy field and into what the samskara wants to share with you. There will be times when you do this meditation with a full-blown triggering situation, and there will also be times when you use it as a way of simply holding the places within that aren't feeling good. It becomes a matter of almost daily hygiene to tend to the places that are inflamed or could potentially flare up. This skill is one that you will take with you for the rest of your life. You will no longer allow samskaras to fester, but instead will gradually release the charge they hold.

DAVID'S STORY

David, a recently retired man in his mid-sixties, shared a triggering experience during a group coaching session. Though he downplayed it, calling it "not that big a deal," he admitted that a recent incident with his younger brother had left him feeling uneasy, and he thought it might serve as a useful example.

David described the situation. His stepdad, who had raised him, was getting old and needed increasing support in his home in Nebraska. His younger brother Tom had sent out a group email to all the siblings to invite them to pitch in. David, who lived in New York City, was not included on the email, but received it as a forward from his younger sister. When David confronted his brother, Tom said that he figured New York was a little too far away for him to be able to help much.

I invited David to pause and sit with that feeling of anger, letting go of the specific details for a moment and noticing where the feeling seemed to settle in his body. After a moment, David placed his hand on his chest and described a heavy, tight sensation. I encouraged him to stay with it, allowing any thoughts or images to arise naturally.

After a quiet moment, David's expression shifted as he muttered, "My brother has always tried to challenge me for firstborn status, to show me I don't really belong." He laughed awkwardly and almost took back his words, but I encouraged him to stay with the feeling, allowing it to be there. I asked if he would explore it a little more to see what might come up.

David closed his eyes and let his mind soften around a memory. "I'm seeing something," he whispered. His voice turned softer, almost childlike, as he continued. "I was around eight years old, and it was our family reunion at the farm. All the cousins were there, but somehow my younger brother—the second oldest, the 'real' son of my stepdad—managed to turn everyone against me. Anytime one of the kids passed by, they'd say things like, 'You're not a Wilson. You're not a real Wilson.' It went on for hours. I felt completely alone and devastated. I tried telling the adults, but they just brushed it off and the teasing only got worse."

Tears filled David's eyes as he continued. "Eventually I couldn't take it anymore and hid in the barn to cry alone. While I was there, they took a big family photo with everyone that was later turned into a painting by a local artist. He had to awkwardly add me in later on, and I never thought it looked realistic. To this day, that painting still hangs in the living room at the farm, a reminder of how I am not a real Wilson."

As he allowed himself to grieve this buried memory, David began to recognize that this old hurt had influenced how he saw his brother's actions for decades. By acknowledging the pain and finally letting himself feel it, he felt a sense of relief and self-compassion.

Exercise

SACRED ROAD MAP MEDITATION

Welcome to your Sacred Road Map Meditation.

This is your sacred time to be with your body, feeling and sensing deep into the wisdom that lives in the body and becoming brilliantly aware of the whole energy field of the body.

As always, start by noticing your breath.

Close your eyes for a moment and just notice how you breathe. Notice where the breath enters easily and where there is constriction in the body. Allow the belly to soften. Invite breath all the way into the lower belly. Feel the movement in the belly when you breathe. Be with that for a minute. Remember how many breaths you typically take per minute. Take that many, with eyes closed.

Let the exhale be an invitation to allow tension to melt out of the energy field of the body.

Let all superficial contractions loosen up and release. Let your body relax into your chair or bed or whatever is supporting you right now.

Now let your body become illuminated with your awareness.

Let all the channels of presence within you open up. Feel into your hands and feet in space and notice details: the temperature of your hands, the feeling of shoes on your feet, or your bare feet. The details will help you become present.

Trace in your mind the outline of your hands and feet and feel into their energy fields. Slowly let your awareness expand from the hands and feet into the arms and legs.

Feel into your face and allow the muscles of your face to soften. Soften around your eyes and forehead.

Let your tongue and throat relax.

Feel into your ears and notice the sense of hearing radiating out. Notice the subtle sound of your own breath inside your ears, any sounds in your immediate space, and any more distant sounds.

Let awareness pour into the whole of your body now, from the lower belly to the solar plexus, chest, and throat. Gradually bring awareness all the way into the core of the energy field of your body. Disperse your awareness very evenly into the whole of the body. Where are your legs? How do they feel? Are they relaxed? How about your arms? Your hands?

Hold awareness in the tips of your fingers, the tips of your toes, the tip of your nose, the top of your head, your earlobes, the soles of your feet, the palms of your hands, and the whole of your face.

Feel into both your arms and your legs now.

Let your belly soften, layer by layer, then even softer. Invite breath into the lower belly. Exhale all the way.

Let your breath be slow and deep. Feel your whole physical self all at once, the whole body and the breath together. Hold the energy field of your body and the rhythm of your breath in your awareness.

Now repeat this simple mantra to the rhythm of your breath: "(*On the inhale*) I am (*on the exhale*) here. I am here, I am here, I am here..." Repeat this for several minutes.

Now you have prepared the vehicle of your body for discovery. Your powers of alertness and sensitivity have been ignited, and you are ready to enter into your inner world to locate and soften what has been held in contraction.

To do so, you can reflect on a recent emotionally charged situation, or simply allow your hands to come to your heart center and bring your full awareness to that space.

Your heart will always tell you which triggering situation needs your attention today.

This is your moment of raw feeling and honesty. You are not looking to be objective right now. You are not trying to be with the facts of the situation.

You are allowing yourself to drop into the feelings that this situation invoked—the subjective feelings that arose in the situation when you were triggered.

You want to spend time with the samskara script, the storyline, the one that you created from the facts, what you made it mean.

Bring the samskara script to mind: what you believe happened and what it meant.

Now repeat this storyline inwardly, in a distilled form.

Tell yourself this painful story now. Speak it out loud if you can, the worst version of the story, the really painful version of this story. Bring it to the surface and feel it in the body. Speak it out loud.

Notice what's happening in your body as you speak these words.

Speak the samskara script out loud. Find the sentence that feels the worst in the body, the sentence that makes your body contract the most.

Let your body feel the resonance of the words.

Now bring awareness into the torso.

Rest your awareness inside your throat. Breathe here. Be here.

Sink into the heart area, the whole chest cavity. Breathe here. Be here.

Feel into the stomach, your solar plexus. Breathe here. Be here.

Sink deeply into the abdomen, your lower belly. Breathe here. Be here.

Hold your awareness in all these parts together.

Now notice where your samskara script is activated. What part of the torso is contracting, reacting most vehemently to the words?

Where does this story show up energetically? Draw your awareness to where this is showing up in the body. Let your hand rest there. Greet this place in the energy field of your body, out loud if you can: "Hi, I feel you. I'm here. I feel you. I notice. I'm here. I want to understand."

Be with this feeling. Notice it.

Keep all your awareness in this area of the body. This feeling is old, is it not? It has been with you for a long time, right?

How old is this feeling?

Let this contracted area show you another time when you felt this way. Go back in time and let your samskara show you prior times when this feeling was activated.

Whatever comes to mind, stay with it. Where are you? How old are you? Who is there? What happened? Let the fullness of that time show itself. Be here. Breathe here.

Feel the pain of this script.

Let the samskara energy show you other times when this feeling was activated. Just be with the contracted energy in the body and notice what other times present themselves. Go back in time and see how old this feeling is.

Watch now, like a movie. How old are you? Who is there? How are others responding to you? What are you making it mean? Speak it out loud. What is the story that is put in place? Feel the contraction, feel the pain.

Is there more?

Give yourself time to experience how often you have felt this feeling.

What did you make this mean?

What did you make this mean about yourself?

What was the message that you internalized?

Draw your awareness very deep into the feeling in the body again. Be here. Breathe.

Hold this place in the body. Feel this injury in your heart-mind energy field (known in yoga as *citta*). Feel this signpost in the sacred road map of the body.

Flood it with your love now. Embrace it with your presence. Be here. Breathe.

Feel it even more deeply.

Get closer. Notice details now. Is this a defined or a diffuse area in the energy field of the body? Is there a color or shape to it?

Is the area dense or fluid?

How is this area responding to your presence?

Is the energy stagnant or is it responding, changing in some way, as you hold it in your awareness? Just notice. There is no right or wrong way of doing this. Your presence is all that is needed.

Breathe and be with this place. Use your mantra: "(*On the inhale*) I am (*on the exhale*) here. I am here, I am here, I am here . . ." Be and breathe.

Surround and penetrate this place with as much presence and love as you can possibly muster.

Notice if your breathing is becoming shallow and recommit to deep, complete inhales and exhales.

Keep noticing where your body may be tensing up in response to being with this place, and let the exhale release all tension from the energy field of the body.

Now gradually let your awareness pull a little away from the epicenter of this contracted energy field.

Start to disperse your energetic awareness into your whole body once more.

Become aware of your hands and your feet, your arms and your legs, the whole of the torso, the throat, jaw, face, ears, scalp, the whole of the head.

Notice your capacity to be grounded in your body.

Breathe deeply while being with the emotional tension within.

Breathe directly into the discomfort, then exhale the discomfort and relax deeply.

Sigh out the tension.

Draw the breath even more deeply into the tight place within, then exhale and release and soften as best you can.

Now slowly open your eyes.

Remain fully grounded and aware of the body, aware of your breath.

Look around you and notice what's there. Let your awareness expand out into the space around you. Notice any sounds in your space and beyond your space. Look around and name what you see nearby and farther away.

Let your awareness expand in all directions: above and below, side to side, front and back.

Let yourself smile softly. Smile at the beauty of your Spirit, loving and holding all your pain, joy, happiness, and sorrow. Smile at your courage to be with it all.

You didn't run away, you didn't lash out, and you didn't numb out. This is beautiful work.

Affirmation Prayer for Locating the Trigger

Divine Love!
Show me with your endless loving light where my pain lies buried within.
Come with me and guide me as I courageously enter the densest, most contracted energy in my body.
Illuminate and love this pained energy that holds story upon story that hurt me along the way.
By the grace of your loving presence, I now hold my deepest pain in so much love and pure empathy as I hear your loving voice speak the truth: "I am here, I love you, I am with you, I will never leave you, and I will hold you now and always."
I fill this place of pain with your vibration of pure loving presence, and I surrender the pain into your Luminous Love that heals one and all, now and always.
So be it and so it is.

Step Five

TRIGGER INQUIRY: UNCOVERING THE SCRIPT

Now you are ready to go a little deeper. Step five on the Heal What Hurts path will teach you how to work with the script(s) that you have located in your body's energy field. You have uncovered the script or story that is activated when you get triggered. Now you will (1) look at where that story comes from so you can heal the original injury with love, and (2) get really clear on how the script has created separation in your relationships and will continue to do so if left in place.

By now you have developed some important skills. You are able to notice when your breath is getting a little shallow or tight. You realize more quickly if you're feeling winded in a situation where you're not exerting yourself or when the body is contracting in some way. You have also gotten better at taking the necessary time and space for yourself, rather than engaging in life-draining drama or a predictable and painful dynamic with the other person.

You may still slip here and there. That's totally normal. Hopefully you've also had the experience of being able to contain the triggered reaction, take space, and not send that text, not make that call, not retaliate, or whatever you would normally do when you engage with a co-triggered person.

You have developed a plan for what you need when you are triggered. You've learned to separate yourself from total overwhelm.

You have learned that your body is a sacred road map that will show you where in your energy field a trigger knot is lodged.

Now we're going to learn how to further extract and make conscious the script that is contained within the trigger knot. We want to get crystal clear on what is fact and what is fiction. In other words, our painful scripts will at times overwhelm us and appear to be factual rather than interpretations of facts. For this you need a pen and paper.

Trigger Inquiry

Your next step on the journey to healing your emotional triggers is to identify what script is being triggered, ignited, and pushed to "play" by a particular situation. Once that script has been identified, you can determine how it invokes certain emotions and feelings in the body.

You want to know how this inner story makes you react and what result you get from that reaction.

You want to slow down the process of being triggered enough that you can extract very precisely the tape that starts running when a certain samskara is activated.

When we begin to detect a glaringly obvious pattern in our storylines, those lines lose some of their powerful grip on our souls. A part of us will stay alert and be able to catch us when we're falling prey to an old storyline yet again.

Let's look at an example from Joyce, a student who attended a workshop of mine. Then we're going to put your own situation into the following Trigger Inquiry Worksheet so you can start to separate facts from your trigger's stories.

Trigger Inquiry Worksheet

Objective Situation (Facts Only): ______________________.

Trigger Script (Your Story): ______________________.

Bodily Sensation: ______________________.

Reaction: ______________________.

Result: ______________________.

Trigger Inquiry Example: Joyce

Joyce was an acclaimed writer and photographer who had just published yet another book that received rave reviews. As had been the case before, she was subsequently invited to speak at an international book fair. She was asked to be on stage, read excerpts from her book, and take questions from the audience. In the past, she had managed to wiggle out of doing this. Once she had even hired an actress to do the reading for her, and another time she claimed she had a scheduling conflict.

But the truth, she confided, was that she was terrified of public speaking. She got sick to her stomach even thinking about it and was already cooking up an excuse for why she could not go to this event either.

"What will happen if you go?" I asked.

"They will realize that I am a fraud," she said. "I won't be able to think straight and I will seem clumsy and nerdy. I can come across as confident in my writing but not in person. I just don't want anyone to see that."

Now, let's separate this out a little bit to get clear on what was real and what was a trigger script that had been activated.

To do this, we will use the Trigger Inquiry Worksheet:

Objective Situation (Facts Only): Joyce was invited to speak at an international book fair and the event planners were waiting for her RSVP.

Trigger Script (Your Story): They will not like me when they see that I am nerdy, clumsy, and not confident.

Bodily Sensation: Anxious contraction in the solar plexus.

Reaction: The first step for Joyce was to drink a big glass of red wine, and then she would get busy coming up with a perfectly plausible excuse for why she wasn't going to be able to make it to the event.

Result: A lost professional opportunity to step into the limelight with her brilliant creative contributions, missing out on meeting other professionals, feeling separated and like she was hiding.

How do we know it was a trigger activation?

Some important clues were the strong bodily reaction and Joyce's overwhelming urge to drink red wine (her numbing agent of choice). She felt undifferentiated anxiety and discomfort in her body and wanted to relax.

When something happens and we want to lash out, numb out, or check out, chances are a trigger has been activated and we are not acting in our own highest interest. Our priority has shifted to the protection of our vulnerability.

I invite you to become skilled at figuring out the storyline in as many of your trigger situations as possible. Practice separating out the raw, objective facts from your story about the situation. The more you are able to separate yourself from the trigger story, the less it will hold power over you and the less real it will feel.

So every time there's a situation that triggers you, first you feel it in your body, you feel it in your breath, you take your space, and then you do your *trigger inquiry*.

Using the Trigger Inquiry Worksheet

Let's take a closer look at the Trigger Inquiry Worksheet using Joyce's example.

Objective Situation (Facts Only): *These are the facts.* No guesses or assumptions are allowed here. Choose something that could be proven in a court of law, like security camera footage. For example, "They will think I am nerdy" is not an objective fact. It is part of the script that was activated by the invitation.

Trigger Script (Your Story): *Highly subjective.* This can feel like facts but is not objectively the truth and could not be proven in a court of law. It is one possible interpretation of a situation that can be challenged and disproven. For example, "They will think I am nerdy" is a fear released from the script, but it can be challenged, because Joyce cannot know this to be true at this point in the chain of events.

Bodily Sensation: The breath and body scan practices from steps one and two will help immensely when you do this step. The more precisely you can locate the feeling of contraction in the body, the closer you are to healing. Numbing agents are not your friend here. They dull and distract you from the very sensations you want to locate and be with. Joyce felt a contraction in her solar plexus, and even thinking about it made her want to drink wine.

Reaction: For Joyce, the first step was indeed drinking a big glass of red wine, and then she got busy coming up with a perfectly plausible excuse for why she wasn't going to be able to make it to the event.

Outcome: *How did the story turn out based on the script, the feelings, and the reaction?* Joyce said she felt shame. Even if she was able to convince the event planners that she was unavailable, *she* knew she wasn't, and her husband also knew she was avoiding being confronted with her fear of public speaking. She was missing out on a step that had the potential to further her career—public reach—not to mention the growth that always follows stepping out of our comfort zone.

Your job is to use this inquiry worksheet with as many triggering situations as possible. As you run your experience through this formula, you will start to notice a pattern in the situations leading to the activation of the trigger scripts. As your trigger scripts are pulled out of the dark corners of your contracted knots in the body, it will become harder for them to overrun you and it will be easier for you to separate yourself from them. That disentanglement from your trigger stories will give you a degree of objectivity that can save you from getting caught up in a whole string of events based on circumstances that may or may not be true.

This is not an easy process. But the more you do it, the more skilled you will become at not confusing factual reality with your story about reality.

This work is the foundation for freeing yourself from emotional triggers that are born out of samskara stories.

How Lizzy Uncovered a Samskara

Lizzy came to me very upset about her friend Sophia, who had stood her up five years earlier, leading to a tear in the relationship. Sophia had recently approached Lizzy about working together on a project, and the old trigger about being stood up was back in full force. Lizzy wasn't sure she would be able to work with Sophia. She experienced tightness in her body even talking about it.

I asked Lizzy to tell me the story of what had happened that led to the breakdown of trust. She said that one summer five years earlier, the two of them had agreed to do yoga on the beach in the morning. Lizzy went to pick up Sophia so they could drive to the beach together. Lizzy was waiting in her car by the side of the road, but her friend failed to appear, so Lizzy got out of the car and went into the family cabin where her friend had been staying for the summer. She entered a flurry of activity. Apparently it was the birthday of one of Sophia's friend's nieces and Sophia was fully engaged in baking a cake. She had forgotten all about the beach yoga date. Sophia apologized but didn't appear to be that disturbed that she had forgotten about yoga. Lizzy, on the other hand, was shaking inside. Even five years later, recalling the moment of realizing her friend had forgotten about their yoga date was deeply upsetting. "I need Sophia to apologize and acknowledge how she let me down!" Lizzy insisted. "Only if she apologizes can I forgive her and feel better about it."

I asked Lizzy to feel into the energy field of her body to sense where the story of being let down this way was showing up. She got all choked up and said she felt tight in her heart and throat. "It's my dad," she said. "He left me with my grandparents in Mexico when I was seven. He left me there for the remainder of my childhood. He took my older brothers with him to the United States and left me behind. I couldn't let go of the anger and pain until my father apologized shortly before he died. When he did, I felt better."

Since we are not inside Lizzy's body, it might be hard to understand how a friend missing yoga on the beach could trigger something as monumental as being abandoned in a foreign country. But for Lizzy, that painful trigger was activated whenever anything smacked of being ignored, dumped, or rejected.

The notion that a sincere apology from someone else is going to guarantee healing is a way of handing the healing power over to some external entity. While an apology *can* contribute to the process of forgiving and moving on, we cannot depend on someone else to comply with our need for one. True healing lies in our own willingness to be present with the tension we feel when we are retriggered.

Exercise

TRIGGER INQUIRY MEDITATION

For this meditation you will want to take notes as I guide you through the Trigger Inquiry Worksheet we just examined.

You will be practicing the fine art of separating out facts from your *trigger script.*

You will learn to look at different situations in your life that cause you to react, to become triggered. You will practice how to separate out what really happened—the objective facts—from the story you are making about it.

Remember, one clue that you are triggered and need to do this work is a *bodily reaction,* a contraction in the energy field somewhere in your body. That is why it's so important that you practice breath and body awareness every single day. If you are stuck in your head, you will miss the clues that you are triggered and will likely proceed to respond to a situation from an unstable inner state—and, more likely than not, there will be numbing agents involved.

Trigger inquiry requires a lot of honesty and self-awareness. It is not easy for the ego to admit that we may not have all the facts of a situation and may indeed be filling in a lot of blanks with samskara scripts.

As always, when you do this work, begin by dropping into an awareness of your breath and your body.

Close your eyes and become aware of your breathing.

Notice the stream of air inside your nose and the rise and fall of your chest and belly.

Might you soften the belly a little more to allow more breath in more deeply?

Sit comfortably in a supported position. Notice the support you are sitting on. Notice your arms and legs. Notice any sounds around you: faraway sounds, sounds closer to you, and the subtle sound of your own body breathing.

Notice how your breath and body awareness helps you become more grounded.

Start noticing the vibrant energy field of your body at this moment.

Life itself gives life to your physical vessel at this moment.

Notice your hands and your feet, vibrantly alive.

Notice how you chose to plant your feet on the earth, however you happen to be sitting right now. Notice your feet. Are your feet bare or are you wearing socks?

Notice your hands. Are they relaxed? Can you feel the energy present in the palms and backs of the hands?

Feel into your fingertips. Mentally trace the outline of your hands and your feet, and feel the space around your hands and feet and the life energy present in them.

Hold that awareness for a moment and, while holding the awareness of your limbs, become more deeply aware of the rhythm of your breath.

Notice if any part of your body is tense, limiting your breath's access to the body.

Breathe fully in and fully out. When the body is deeply relaxed, the breathing rhythm slows down and you can drop into a slower and more mindful way of breathing.

Stay very alert while noticing the sensation of being very alive in your hands and feet.

Let that sensation spread into the whole of the body, filling your legs and arms, then the torso, inside and out, front and back, left side and right side.

Relax your shoulders, throat, chin, and lips. Feel the subtle stream of air inside the nose. Soften around the eyes and nose and soften the forehead.

Feel into your ears now. Maintain this grounded, vibrant presence in the body.

With your eyes open, maintain that slower, deeper cadence of the breath.

Look around you and name what you see.

Slowly turn your head in both directions. Let your eyes rest for a moment on various objects around you.

Feel the temperature around you and notice any scents around you.

Bring your awareness to your heart center. You may bring your hands to this space in a prayer gesture or lay them gently on your chest.

Then inwardly ask that any situation where you were triggered arise now for you to take a closer look.

Start by stating what happened.

You are not yet going deep into your feelings around the situation. You will be doing that when you do your trigger inquiry in a moment.

For now you are harvesting the details of the triggering situation in a very factual, objective way.

Allow your heart to help you recall a recent situation where you felt triggered.

Remember who was there. Where were you? What happened?

Now jot down the facts. In Lizzy's case, she would simply state that Sophia had missed their yoga date and had baked a cake instead.

Do not, at this point, go into how the situation made you feel or how it made you react.

Stating dry, objective facts can be a little difficult, because we tend to color and overlay our memories with our stories about them. For example, Lizzy might say, "Sophia didn't care about our yoga date," but that is not a fact. That is an interpretation of the situation and belongs in the *trigger story*.

Do your best here to cut to the bone of what happened.

If there were other people involved, as is usually the case when we're triggered, write down only what they actually said or did, and only if it's purely factual.

Don't assign motives. Don't make assumptions.

Get really precise about it and be brief. You are not soliciting support or justifying your reaction, but just stating what happened. The other person(s) would fully agree with your description of the situation.

This is your ***Objective Situation.*** Write it down.

Now you get to be subjective. Petty. Have charged opinions about what happened. Judgments. Even anger and resentment, sadness, frustration, jealousy. Allow yourself to feel that. Notice where those feelings show up in the energy field of the body.

Write it down. "She is so thoughtless. She shouldn't . . ." "She clearly feels this or that about me." "She always . . ." "She never . . ." "They definitely are . . ."

Get mad for a moment. No one has to see this. Just let it rip.

Then pause and see if you can capture the whole tirade in a sentence or two. Feel into your body. The stronger the energetic response in the body, the more accurate your sentence is.

This is your ***Trigger Script.*** Write it down.

Now repeat your trigger script softly to yourself and see where the body reacts to it. Scan your body and see what part of the torso seems to react when it hears this script spoken aloud. Describe in detail the bodily sensation: the location, size, shape, and any other descriptors that fit this feeling in the energy field of the body. How is your breathing rate? Are you able to breathe deeply and calmly?

This is your ***Bodily Sensation.*** Write it down.

Now you need to be very real about what you do in this circumstance.

You know you are triggered. Your body and breath are clearly showing you that.

You have extracted the painful trigger script.

What is your greatest urge when you speak this script out loud and feel the sensations in your body?

My typical trigger reaction is to lash out, numb out, or check out.

What is your pattern? How do you react to the trigger script? It may not always be the same, but you will likely find that you have a typical way of reacting.

Ask yourself, "When I hear the words of my trigger script and I feel the bodily sensations, I really want to..."

That is your ***Reaction.*** Write it down.

In your mind's eye, do that thing you do when you are triggered, or recall a time when you did that thing. What was the *result* of that action? What happened or didn't happen as a direct consequence of your trigger reaction?

Write that down. This is your ***Result.***

Now that you have slowed down your process and become clearer on how your triggers play into your interpretation of any situation in which you find yourself triggered, you can question the trigger story.

Ask yourself this: "Is my trigger story 100 percent true? Can I absolutely know that this story is the truth and nothing but the truth? Might I be able to write down three examples of my trigger story not being true in this situation?"

Write down three examples of your samskara story not being true. Notice how the energy field of your body responds to your three examples of the samskara story not being true.

What might be your reaction if it was born out of this sensation in the body?

What might be the result if your reaction and actions were different?

Use your imagination. Now picture the same situation, but imagine a more loving, grounded script playing out instead. Ask yourself: "What else might be true here? Is there another way to see this? How might I respond from love rather than fear?"

What if the script that has been running—the one that interprets others' words or actions as personal, disrespectful, or rejecting—was no longer the only story available? If that painful meaning wasn't the only lens, how else might you see this moment? Is there a sliver of possibility that the other person isn't a villain but is simply acting from their own pain, confusion, or limits?

Could it be that…

- They didn't mean to hurt you—they were just overwhelmed or distracted?
- They were doing the best they could with the tools they had?
- Their actions weren't about you at all?

This isn't about excusing harmful behavior. It's about softening the grip of an old story and allowing space for a different kind of truth to emerge—one that brings more peace to your body, your relationships, and your life.

We are not abandoning the trigger script here. We want to explore *why* that script is there in the first place. We want to find the pained place within that holds onto this painful version of reality.

Now that you've examined your current emotional script, the next step is to gently uncover where it began. The body remembers. The pain we feel now often points to a deeper origin. Let's go there next—with loving compassion.

Affirmation Prayer for Feeling Deeply Loved

Divine Love!

I call upon your wisdom light and compassionate light to fill my awareness now

As I seek to understand what is really going on inside of me when I react.

Help me stay in my witnessing consciousness inspired only by your loving light.

I seek to know myself, understand myself, while staying in the deep, abiding compassion that you have for me and fill me with.

Help me now to separate out from the pain that is triggered and help me see how I am replaying old stories and engaging in patterns that I have the power, through your loving grace within me, to break and be free from.

Now and forever.

So be it and so it is.

Step Six

THE ORIGIN OF THE TRIGGER STORY

There is always a reason that you resort to an *out*. The pain that is being triggered is not just about what's happening in the present; it's also reactivating the contracted trigger knot from pain previously experienced but not processed. Step six on the Heal What Hurts path will guide you to understand where the script originated and gradually replace the trigger-produced beliefs with loving ones that empower you.

There are two layers to this work:

1. We want to continue to challenge the validity of the trigger script in any current situation. When we are triggered, our thinking can become very black-and-white: "You always..." or "You never..." Is the situation possibly more complex than the trigger script would have you believe?
2. We want to feel deeper into the energy field of the body and explore how old this script is. When was the first time you remember feeling this way? Regardless of what arises here—whether it's a whole

> story from the past, a fleeting memory, or no distinct memory—the wounded parts of ourselves always need to be held with compassion. When we hold a wounded piece of ourselves in great love and compassion so as to melt and ultimately release the contraction, it loses its charge and ceases to fire off the same script over and over.

As we progress, this work must be done more or less formally every time we feel triggered if we want to heal at the root level. We will not be able to release the grip of the current experience if we don't challenge the validity of the trigger story that sits like a belief embedded in the body and we will likely remain in conflict with the stand-in villain. That is the current person who reminds us energetically of a primary caretaker failing us. And we will very likely call in another version of the same painful scenario if we don't pull the projection back into its source in the energy field of the body and then work to soften and release the contracted energy.

As the trigger gradually loses its tight grip, we make room for a new story based on new beliefs. We become free to co-create our lives instead of living out a painful story again and again.

When a trigger script has been activated, it's like you are viewing a given person or situation through that particular filter, and there is not much room for a more nuanced view of the person or situation.

Emily, a young nurse who came to a Heal What Hurts workshop, was convinced that her superior did not appreciate her work. She shared, "My manager makes me feel like I can't do anything right. She is always correcting me and never praising me."

I asked, "Is that always true? Has your manager never expressed appreciation for your work? Has she ever indicated that you are a qualified person?"

Often we can shoot holes in how we apply our trigger script in a given situation, but only if we are willing to take the time to identify the script or the assumption we are making. (Remember, the words *always* and *never* are clues that we are triggered.) We want to bring the script we are running out into the light and write it down.

In this case, Emily was actually able to think of quite a few examples of her manager praising her work and appreciating her as a person. This allowed her to feel past the current story and go into the energy field of her body and notice what part of her body contracted in reaction to her initial story: "She never appreciates me and is always correcting me." Not surprisingly, that was an old childhood feeling that she was superimposing on her current work situation. Bringing loving awareness to the trigger knot in her body and at least somewhat releasing it allowed her to step into a more adult relationship with her manager at work.

When we know what a painful script sounds like, we can counter it. Not all at once and not overnight, but gradually, we will be able to stay present and awake enough when it starts to play. We will notice that contracted feeling in the energy field of the body and go, "Uh-oh, here we go." Then the script starts to play within, very often some version of, "I am not loved. I am not safe. I don't belong."

Getting to Know What the Script Sounds Like

At this point in the process, you likely have a pretty good sense of something that happened when you were much younger that keeps playing out in your adult relationships. I hope you have become better at not judging or shaming yourself for the triggered feeling—or even the *out* that you find yourself resorting to. When appropriate and when you feel emotionally safe, you may have even been able to communicate with the person who triggered you. If you vulnerably confide the old hurt that makes you react strongly to a certain behavior and the subsequent *out* reaction that comes from a wounded place within, chances are you will discover that the person you are in a triggered conflict with has also been triggered in some way by you—that you are *both* busy telling yourselves stories about the other person's motives.

Knowledge Is Power

When you know what your typical painful script sounds like and how it's been operating inside of you, you have the option of creating a new script. You *can* become a more conscious co-creator of your reality and your experience in relationships. In this step, you'll begin to replace the old script by working with a new affirmation and a visualization to help anchor a more loving and empowered internal narrative. Be aware, however, that as you decide to implement a new script, the old beliefs held in your trigger knots will protest and contract in response. When this happens, you know what to do: Hold the contracted energy with your compassionate presence. Speak to the place within with words and listen to it fire off its negative beliefs. Just keep bathing the contracted knot with patient, steady love: "I am here. I love you. I've got you." You will notice the contraction start to soften, and gradually the negative beliefs will become less powerful.

The Healing Cure Is Always Loving Presence

Most trigger scripts that I have been privy to in students, clients, and myself are all variations on the same themes, what humans fear the most: *I am not loved. I am not safe. I don't belong*. When you become convinced that this trigger script is not the truth, you can gradually replace it with positive affirmations that produce the result in your life that you do want. The problem with manifesting and affirmations is that the underlying negative trigger scripts often have not been made conscious and hence cannot be challenged and purged.

In the New Script Meditation that I offer for this step later in this chapter, you will be invited to set a new vision, to reprogram your inner stories while being infinitely patient with the triggers that are still in the process of softening and releasing.

As you shift your vision, your words, your script, you will start to attract situations that match the new script—sometimes with lightning speed. You will start to draw in new situations, and new dynamics between you and others will arise.

My client Sandra was unhappy with what she perceived as her boyfriend's frugality, which she felt bordered on being miserly. Whenever she perceived him as not treating her with generosity, she felt depressed and unlovable. I asked her to tune into her body instead of challenging her boyfriend to be more generous with her. She became focused and still inside. A contracted knot showed up on the left side of her belly button, and I asked her to just sit with it. After a few minutes, she started talking: "It's about my mom. She was with a boyfriend after my dad died, and while they were together for years, she felt neglected and never fully chosen."

Sandra was feeling her mother's belief in her body—a belief that she was not worthy of being treated with generosity and commitment. As Sandra sat with the contraction in her body, we called upon the Divine to beam the knot with loving compassion and stated the intention to release and let go of this painful belief so it would stop manifesting as reality. We ended with a positive affirmation: "I am worthy of being showered with love and generosity." The knot slowly softened and felt less charged. This new and much more expansive belief could take root in Sandra's energy field because the negative belief had lost its charge and was on its way out.

The next time Sandra checked in with me, she told me that the day after the session, her boyfriend had surprised her with a gesture of love and big generosity. Furthermore, she said she had realized that even before our session there had been plenty of generous gestures, but it had been hard for her to take them in because she was seeing them through the lens of the negative belief.

The beliefs and stories we carry within are powerful. They are essentially unconscious affirmations or even prayers that are running 24/7, and we must uproot the ones that hurt us and others. It's all about feeling the contracted knots in the body where they live. Words are prayers, invocations, magic. Essentially, our words—whether in the form of thoughts, spoken words, or written words—manifest in the world. In yoga, we think of the whole universe as coming into being through the primordial sound of Om.

Throughout history, words have been known to be incredibly powerful. We simply cannot create the life we dream of if we do not uproot the tense knots that carry painful stories and beliefs.

You Have the Power to Speak Good into Your Life

The good news is that you *can* speak something new and better into being. Pause for a moment. Consider what you currently have in your life that you spoke into being, something that wasn't there until you decided to give it your energy and make it so. Everything in your life has at some point come into manifestation. Some of it was the result of your careful, intentional manifestation of something you really wanted. Now it's here. Congratulations! This is the power of manifestation at work, co-creation. So take responsibility for your words and even your thoughts.

From now on and for as long as you live, be aware of what you're speaking into the world, whether it's with your thoughts, spoken words, or written words. You need to extract the trigger scripts and long-held beliefs, or you can't challenge them. And once you know what they are, it's your responsibility to prevent them from taking over and tainting your life and the lives of others. At any given time, take a look at your life experience, the whole tableau, and ask yourself, "How did my beliefs contribute to this?" Write it down, what beliefs were at play to create all this, the good, the bad, and the ugly. Take one belief at a time and notice where in the body you are reacting/contracting in the energy of that belief.

The meditation I will guide you through for this step will invite you to create scripts that are soothing, calming, exciting, and creative new ways for you to be in the world. You can speak your affirmations inside your head over and over, and you can speak them out loud during the meditation. You can speak them out loud whenever you have privacy, like when you are sitting alone in the car. You can write them in your journal, and you can even tell a trusted friend whom you know would hold this new story with and for you. In short, you declare it, declare it, declare it, repeatedly.

What will happen over time is that the old script, the old sad story that has tripped you up so many times, will be the one that sounds like a lie. You will be increasingly aware when the trigger knot is stirring and the old script is starting to run. You will realize that you are now wearing a certain pair of glasses through which you are viewing a certain situation or person. If you are in a state of reaction to the trigger, you will not be able to see completely clearly. But if you can recognize that you are triggered and have the ability to extract and name the story, you will be out from under its total tyranny. If you can seize that moment when the trigger script is apparent to find the trigger knot in the body, you have the opportunity to transform the energy. From that perspective, being triggered is not something to be avoided; it's a sacred moment to bring loving, compassionate presence to a place inside where energy does not flow freely. As long as you can do less *out* and more *in*, you will begin to notice tangible shifts in your life experience.

You might ask, "How do I know whether I'm having a strong, valid intuition that someone is out to get me or it's just a trigger story acting up?" That's a good question, because both your intuition and your trigger stories operate inside the energy field of your body. The medicine is always the same: Locate the contracted energy and douse it with loving presence while gently hushing up the story that wants to be fed. The more you do that, the more accurate your perception of reality will be.

Years ago I was going to a function at my kids' school shortly after getting divorced. I was sitting in my car in the parking lot, dreading walking in by myself. I was certain that everyone would judge me, would not like me, and would not want to talk to me. I pictured having to sit alone. As I sat there and breathed the fear in my belly, I was momentarily revisited by a time in seventh grade when the boy who used to like me turned on me.

I don't even remember why, but from my point of view, he made it his business to get other kids on his side, and for a period of a few weeks I felt judged, lonely, and not liked.

I recognized that I had created this painful story about the other parents at the school, and I prayed for help in manifesting something different from my triggered expectation. Sitting right there in my car, I rewrote in my mind the miserable little story I'd concocted about the other parents judging me. Then I walked into the school.

I was met with so much warmth and kindness that I almost cried. My initial story couldn't have been further from my actual experience. But what if I had walked into the school with the original negative story in my mind? Would I have had a completely different experience?

Exercise

MEDITATION TO DISCOVER THE ORIGIN OF THE TRIGGER: COMPASSIONATE SITTING WITH THE SEED OF THE PAIN

Welcome to the Meditation to Discover the Origin of the Trigger, an invitation for what lives in your body to communicate to your conscious self and an invitation for *you*, your more conscious self, to really listen to what is happening in the body when you are emotionally triggered.

It's deeply uncomfortable to be triggered by something or someone, and most people run away from that feeling—by lashing out, numbing out, or checking out.

This is an invitation to go inward with compassion and really feel and understand where the trigger comes from—not simply changing the words around it or trying to get someone else to change their behavior, but understanding with deep empathy and a willingness to feel and be with the parts of you that hurt the most.

To fully tune into what lives in the energy field of the body, you must become fully present in the energy field of the body. We have been trained to live in the head, in the intellect. Most of us are somewhat numb in the body.

So before we can begin the deep work of embracing, loving, and healing the samskaras—the triggered energies within the body—we must first become as present as we possibly can.

I invite you to close your eyes. You can be seated or resting on your back.

The first step is to become a lot more aware of your own breathing. Allow the inhale to be just a little bit deeper. Guide the inhale into the lower abdomen and let the exhale complete itself. Notice how there might be a little bit more air that you could simply release and let go of at the very bottom of your exhale.

There's a softening in the body. The inhale is a little longer. The exhale is a little bit longer as well. The mind has already quieted down significantly simply by shifting the awareness to the breath.

As you become increasingly aware of the breath, you're starting to sync up with your Spirit Self. The temporary thoughts are releasing their stronghold on your awareness.

Now remain aware of your breath. Let it be comfortable. You're not straining to breathe more deeply. You're just letting your breaths be full and rich and voluminous. Allow your whole being to really experience the relaxation that comes with a deep exhale.

Notice the way the breath feels inside your nose. Perhaps there is a sound inside your ears—a subtle sound of your own breath.

Stay focused on the rhythm of your breath and simultaneously draw your awareness into your heels. Feel into the tops of the feet, the soles of the feet, and the toes. Now trace in your mind your ankles, your shin bones, and your calves. Sense and feel into the presence of awareness and life force.

Feel into your lower legs, your ankles, your feet, and your toes. Now slowly let the sense of awareness expand up through the knees and thighs.

You might even picture the awareness as light—as though you are gradually illuminating the energy field of your body with your awareness, essentially spiritualizing the energy field of your body.

Let the sense of presence and awareness spread from the thighs into the hip sockets, the pelvic bowl, the lower abdomen, and the lower back. Soften the belly. Relax the belly.

Let the awareness now fill the mid-back and the whole solar plexus, belly button, and stomach area—relaxing ever more deeply as more awareness fills the body.

Let the awareness now expand up into the upper back and the shoulder blades—the right shoulder blade and the muscles around it, beneath it, and above it, the whole right shoulder blade, and the right shoulder—releasing and relaxing.

Now bring awareness into the left shoulder blade. Feel the left shoulder, the whole left side of the chest—relaxing, softening.

Now send the awareness down through both arms: from the shoulders into the upper arms, the elbows, the forearms, the wrists, the hands, the backs of the hands, the thumbs, index fingers, middle fingers, ring fingers, and pinkies. Send the awareness through the palms of the hands, the backs of the hands, and the tips of all ten fingers.

Slowly zoom in on this area with great loving care and communicate to this part of the energy field of your body.

Let the awareness expand up through the back of the neck and the throat. Relax the sides of the neck. Let your jaw relax and fill with awareness.

Relax your chin and your lips, your tongue and your teeth, the nasal cavities, the eyeballs, eyelashes, eyelids, eyebrows. Relax the space between the eyebrows and the whole of the forehead. Relax the right ear, the wrinkles and folds of the right ear, the left ear, the wrinkles and folds of the left ear.

Soften around the whole scalp—the back of the head, the sides of the head, the top of the head. Feel every hair follicle relaxing.

Now hold maximum awareness in the entire energy field of your body. Maximum awareness in the whole energy field of the body.

And now draw your awareness into the torso. Feel deeply into the torso: from the throat through the chest area, the solar plexus, and the belly button. Feel into the lower abdomen. Feel into the whole torso.

And now notice where in the torso the energy seems to be flowing less fluidly—with some degree of stagnation, stuckness, or contraction.

Let your body guide you into the most contracted area in the energy field of your torso. Say to it:

I am here to love you.
I'm here to get to know you.
I'm here to listen.
I'm here to hold you, to be with you.

I've got you.
I sense you.

Now simply *be* with the felt sensation. Do your best not to go into any kind of story about the sensation. With your capacity for presence, surround and penetrate, hold, and be with this contracted energy.

Notice what happens to the energy. How does the energy respond to your presence, to your kind words? Say to it:

I'm here.
I feel you.
I notice you.
I want to know you.
I want to feel you.
I want to hold you.
I'm here and I love you.
I'm here and I've got you.
I'm here. I'm with you.

Now in this state of simply being with the contracted energy…

Notice how this is likely a familiar feeling—one that has shown itself at other times in your life. Ask your body, this area in your body: How old is this feeling? When is the first time you remember having this feeling? Stay with the feeling in the body and allow this place inside to show you what is contained here. What does this feeling remind you of?

Whatever memory arises, just be with it and notice as many details as you can. How old do you think you were when you first experienced this feeling? Who was there? Where are you? Allow details to emerge if they want to.

If there is no memory, just be with the feeling. Just hold it and be with it. Stay with the contracted feeling and notice how it responds to your inquiry, to your presence.

If there is a memory, go even closer. Be in the memory. It may start out like a photograph. Then let it become a movie. And then step into the movie set and see what you remember.

Ask yourself again: Who is there? How are you feeling in that situation? Are the feelings of anyone around you tainting your feelings? Stay with the felt sensation in the body. Is it shifting, contracting more? Relaxing? Notice the energy and keep sending soothing words to this contracted place inside:

I am here.
I've got you.
I want to hear your story.

Notice if you have the urge to yawn, sigh, or cry. Allow your body to guide what needs to happen. Stay with the sensation. Visualize the sensation being embraced by light as you quietly whisper or inwardly state:

I am here.
I love you.
I know this hurts and I am right here with you.

Don't force anything. Just be with whatever arises with great patience and great understanding. Communicate yet again:

I'm here and I love you.
I'm here and I'm with you.
I love you.

Stay in the space. See what else shows itself as you stay close to and interested in this sensation in the body. Stay so close that you notice any little shift in the energy while you simply stay with whatever arises as you hold and stay present with this memory, this felt sensation in the body.

Trust that anything that comes up is relevant. Don't try to analyze it. Just notice.

Stay with the sensation, the most dominant sensation in the energy field of the body, as you allow the memories contained within this contraction to become clearer. Shower this part of your energy field with love yet again:

I love you and I'm here.
I'm with you.

Notice every little subtle shift in the energy in the body. How does the body respond to your presence? What else would your body like to show you? You can ask it:

What else would you like to show me about this?

Notice any feelings that arise. If there are tears, let them flow, but don't go into the story. Stay with the felt sensation in the body.

The mind is still. All the awareness is in the energy field of the body.

Ask your body now:

What makes this feeling worse?
When does this feeling show up?

Stay with the physical sensation and simply notice any shifting in the energy. Does it stay in the same place? Does the contraction feel like it's tightening up, loosening, or staying the same?

I am here and I love you.

Now ask this place within:

Is there something else you would like to show me?

This could be in either pictures, words, or sensations in the body.

Now communicate to this place within yet again:

I love you and I'm here.

And I will be your friend now and stay with you and listen to you and be there for you, especially when uncomfortable feelings arise in the energy field of the body.

I will be right there.

I will come back often and check, and I will heed your call when you need me.

Now slowly start to expand your awareness back into the whole energy field of the body, dispersing once more your awareness very evenly around the body.

Notice how it's easier this time around, as all the channels of awareness are open.

Notice the breath and take a deep breath in and exhale audibly through your mouth. Do that two more times. Really allow tension to release through the yawn. Take a deep breath in—and even bigger. Let it be audible. Let it come from a deep place within the body.

Return to what feels like natural breath now. Feel the whole of the body.

If you are sleepy and would like to stay, take a nap, or continue to meditate, you can simply turn off this recording and do so. If you're ready to come out, let it be slow.

If you're lying on your back, roll to the right side and then slowly push yourself up to seated.

Now scan the body one more time to take a deep imprint of what it feels like to be this present in the body. Quietly promise your body to be more present more of the time, conducting mini body scans all day long—regularly, lovingly, giving presence and awareness to the whole of the body.

Then ever so slowly, open your eyes, still staying present in the body.

Let yourself move on with your day with this increased awareness in the energy field of the body, vowing to come back to this practice often—out of deep self-love for the body.

Affirmation Prayer for Healing the Original Wound

Dear God, loving presence, luminous light within,

By the grace and healing power of your light and your eternal love for me, I call for profound healing of the original injury that caused my body to contract and hold onto pain.

I now allow your love to surround and penetrate the contracted energy inside of me and to lift me to ever higher ground in love, in life, in my work.

I now allow the highest frequency of companions, events, and experiences to flow into my life.

Miracles here in my life. Goodness here in my life. Grace here in my life. All is well.

I open myself up fully and completely to your luminous love and light to fill my being and guide me on my path.

So be it and so it is.

Exercise

NEW SCRIPT MEDITATION

Let yourself drop into your body and breath. Become present. Let your breath guide you into the present moment. Let your belly soften and become more receptive to a deeper breathing pattern.

Let the exhale draw out any tension that is in your body. Let your body become relaxed. Listen to the subtle sound of your breath. Feel your breath inside your nose: the coolness of the inhale, the warmer exhale.

Notice where your body feels a little tight, and release. Soften your shoulders. Soften the little muscles around the eyes. Let your jaw relax. Feel into your feet. Let all the little muscles of the feet relax. Feel into your hands. Let your hands become soft and relaxed.

Let awareness expand from your hands and feet into your limbs and then your torso. Notice the cadence of your breath, the rise and fall of your belly and chest. The mind is quieting down as you become more present in your body and more aware of your breath.

All is well. You are in this moment, breathing, safely held in the arms of the earth. Relax into the cradle of the space you are in. Feel the peace of this moment. Relax into this moment in the world. Relax even more deeply.

Feel into the body now. Allow any remaining tension and contraction to soften and melt away. Soft, open heart. Spacious heart.

Let your awareness drop into the heart center. Pose the question to your heart, "What do you need, dear heart?" What would be really wonderful? Whether it's in regard to a specific relationship or something more general, ask yourself what you truly need.

What would you ideally feel like? What would be the wonderful version of your situation or your relationship? Let yourself state it as a wish. What do you wish for? "I really wish that..."

And now, if it *were* like that, how would you feel? You are not attempting to change someone else here but are imagining yourself in a peaceful place regardless of what everyone else is doing or saying. What would that feel like and look like?

What would it feel like inside of you if this situation or relationship were healthy? Who would you be? Can you formulate that into something like a sentence, an affirmation? You can speak it in the future tense to begin with and then we will shift it: "I really wish that..."

If what arises inside is the feeling that someone else is doing or being something counter to that wish, ask yourself, "What belief might I be carrying that allows me to remain in a dynamic with someone I perceive as treating me this way?" Find the belief by formulating how you perceive this other person's engagement with you: "He/she/they are doing x, y, z to me—or they are failing to do x, y, z..." Notice *where* in your body you feel this script. Speak it out loud a few times. Feel the full force of the pain this belief is inflicting.

You are speaking this painful belief out loud to tease out the contracted trigger knot that is associated with this story. Make it really obvious where the contracted energy is in the body by wording the painful belief with complete honesty.

For example, a female client of mine realized she was holding the belief "He'll never leave his wife for me." At first she assumed the belief was her own, but when she sat with the feeling of that belief lodged like a contraction in her body, she had a tearful memory of her mother. As a child, she had watched her mom yearn for a boyfriend who had never pursued a divorce, even though he had been long estranged from his wife. That painful emotional imprint had embedded itself in her system. As she let herself fully feel the memory and the belief inside it, she wept—and the contraction softened. A year later, she was happily married to the man she loved. When she released the belief that it would never happen, something different was able to manifest for her and her partner.

We co-create our reality through the beliefs we carry—especially the unconscious ones. When we begin to question them and let go of the ones that no longer serve us, our outer lives begin to reflect the shift within.

When you speak the painful belief out loud, do you feel the contracted knot? Then release and let go of the story. Reduce the experience to the contracted knot in your body. Just sit with this painful sensation of contraction in the body. Be as precise as you can. Be a scientist, a surgeon even, looking very closely through your microscope, relaxing the examined area as best you can. Then say gently to this contracted, pained knot: "I am here. I love you. I've got you. I am just going to be right here, holding you, noticing you, radiating loving compassion into you."

Beam this loving medicine of presence into the knot. Be with it, notice it, sense it. It may be really uncomfortable to allow this contracted pain to become so visible, so obvious. Call upon the Divine Love within you: "Divine Love, be with me. Radiate loving light into my pain. Soothe this knot in my energy. Radiate loving light into this frozen knot and let me receive the healing energy of your presence. I allow Divine Love in, fully in. I surrender to the healing power of divine, loving presence within. I soften my body and receive Divine Love. Goodness here. Grace here. Divine Love here. In me. Now and always."

Allow yourself to bathe in this energy of ever more Divine Love entering the pain. Allow yourself to feel the pain that is softening and opening and allowing Divine Love deeply in, like the warm sun slowly melting a hard piece of ice.

Now let's convert that wish into a present-tense affirmation. Take the feeling you are wishing to feel, for example, "I wish I felt peaceful."

The present-tense affirmation is "I am so happy and grateful now that, by the power of the Divine within me, I am peaceful inside."

We are not in anyone else's business. We are manifesting an inner state of being that does not depend on another person's chosen behavior. "I am so happy and grateful now that, by the power of the Divine within me, I am peaceful inside."

Now match your affirmation to the cadence of your breath: "(*On the inhale*) I am so happy and grateful now that, (*on the exhale*) by the power of the Divine within me, I am peaceful inside." You can choose to take several breaths for each affirmation. Just find a soft rhythm.

Or you might distill your affirmation down to something like this: "(*On the inhale*) By the power of the Divine within me, (*on the exhale*) I am peaceful inside," or whatever your chosen feeling is. Notice if there is any part of your body's energy field that contracts against the words, protests the words. If so, direct the words of your affirmation, like an energetic laser beam, directly into that area of the body.

Let it be okay if there is a little part of you that is not so sure about your affirmation yet, that doesn't believe it could be that easy. Let yourself sit in the energetic shower of these words: "I am so happy and grateful now that I am filled with …" "By the power of the Divine, I am now filled with …" You can play around with how you say it.

Feel the quality of your chosen feeling as an energy inside your body. Let this positive feeling fill your body. Imagine the feeling made of light, and let the light fill you up. Let every cell in your body soak up the feeling of this positive feeling.

Focus in particular on any samskara energies that are acting up in protest against this energy, and just hold the contraction with the positive feeling energy. Sit in the shower of this beautiful energy and come back to it often.

You can also choose a more specific counter-script born directly out of your samskara script. For example, "I don't fit in and I am not loved" would become "I fit in and I belong." You may encounter more resistance when you come at the samskara script like that, but it is still very effective, and over time you will no longer believe the negative samskara script.

The old script may act up for a while, but when you feel that familiar energy in your body indicating that you are not safe, don't belong, and are not loved, you will gradually learn to patiently say, "That is not true. You are loved. You are safe. You belong. I am loved. I am safe. I belong."

Affirmation Prayer for a New Script

Dear God, loving presence, luminous light within,

Inspired by your light and your eternal love for me, I set in motion a divinely inspired script for my life path.

I now allow your love to guide me to ever higher ground in love, in life, in my work.

I now allow the highest frequency of companions, events, and experiences to flow into my life. Miracles here in my life. Goodness here in my life. Grace here in my life. All is well. I open myself up fully and completely to your luminous love and light to fill my being and guide me on my path.

So be it and so it is.

Step Seven
FORGIVENESS

You have come a long way doing this beautiful, courageous, and self-loving practice. If you have practiced the previous steps, you have likely noticed a shift in your capacity to maintain a steadier state internally as well as externally—in your relationships and in your life experience in general. Yet there is still some cleanup work to do.

Step seven on the Heal What Hurts path is an invitation to release anger and resentment from your body. Although such feelings may be justified, it is time to let them go, because they harden you against life. Forgiveness is the process of shedding the burden of grievances and becoming available to the miracle of life flowing through you.

Forgiving Releases Blocked Life Force

Most of us have spent our whole life—if not previous lifetimes as well—projecting our trigger scripts out into the world. With our projections we cast someone else in the role of the villain, usually a stand-in for a person from our childhood who failed to meet our needs. Whether in the distant past, in a past life, or in the present moment, the villain we create with our projections activates this painful place within us. That villain is probably still stuck in our energy field, assuming the form of a grudge, blame, or judgment we cast toward others.

Your villains likely stem from more recent events as well as someone who played that role in your childhood. Whoever it is, they are likely to be someone you perceive to have failed to treat you with love and compassion at a crucial time. Now it's time to release that person from the role they have played in your life. Now it's time to forgive them.

If we encounter strong resistance to forgiving, we're going to miss this step. If we miss forgiving, we miss an opportunity to move on into the present unfolding around us. This is the time for the Forgiveness Meditation presented later in this chapter. But before we get to the Forgiveness Meditation, we need to talk about what forgiveness is and is not.

Forgiveness Does Not Mean Condoning

Forgiveness in the context of this process is not asking you to condone hurtful behavior, nor is it telling your villain or any other agent of harm that what happened was okay. Forgiveness is a practice of releasing the contraction of resentment from your energy field so you can breathe freely again.

Forgiveness is an ongoing *practice*. It is a practice of releasing and letting go of a judgment. When you condemn someone, you energetically lock yourself in with that person, and that impacts you. A portion of your energy field is in contraction, and prana cannot flow freely through it. Holding onto your judgment causes a blockage that restricts all your other behaviors. We want to clear that person's energy from our energy field by releasing them.

Again, when we forgive another person, we are not saying, "It's okay that you hurt me." Hurting another person is never okay, and it's never your fault that someone hurt you. If a trigger was instilled and ended up playing out in hurtful ways, that's not because you deserved to be hurt. But through your powerful, divine, loving presence, you *do* have the power to release it and become free.

A trigger caused by prior hurt that is now stuck in the energy field may very well have contributed to attracting hurtful people and events, but that doesn't mean you caused the hurt or deserved it. It might mean you may have carried low expectations of how much love and respect you deserve, and it might mean you didn't walk away from a hurtful situation sooner because you didn't know you deserved better.

We can change that now. When you come into full love for yourself, you *will* walk away if you are being mistreated. When you come into full love for yourself, you will *not* stay in an abusive situation because you fear being alone. You will *never* be alone when you come into full love for yourself. You will not give away your power when you come into full love for yourself. You will not need anyone else to maintain your state of love for yourself.

Self-Love Is the Antidote to Codependency

Self-love does not mean that you will not attract and enjoy loving and supportive relationships but rather that you will gradually disentangle yourself from codependency. You will stay in your own business and you will attract and be attracted to people who are fully present in their own lives and don't need you to feel complete.

During this step of healing your emotional triggers, you are invited to release the anger and resentment you hold in your body toward someone else. Any anger or resentment within you is hurting *you*, and you are coming into so much love for yourself that you are not willing to carry anger in your body any longer. Anger is a toxic energy that blocks the flow of your life.

In the past and possibly even in your life right now, someone likely did or said something that wasn't loving or even kind. It might be that this person's woundedness hooked into your woundedness, and that created reactive behavior in each of you. The two of you were likely co-triggered. Or maybe you were the innocent victim of a jerk and it really hurt. That's totally possible too.

Unforgiveness Is a Poison in Your Body

We don't have to understand why the other person did what they did, and we don't have to wait around for them to feel sorry, but we *do* need to forgive them so we can move on and be free inside. Holding a grudge is a very toxic energy. I once heard a teacher say that if you don't forgive, it's like taking poison and hoping the other person dies.

If you are building any kind of relationship (romantic, platonic, working, etc.) with someone, you will probably step on each other's toes once in a while. If you are not aware of this, the grudges may well pile up and become lodged like trigger knots in your energy field. The resentment will be easily reignited when the circumstances are right. Any progress the two of you might have made in terms of building trust will be wiped out time and again as the trespasses of the past spew out of this constantly reactivated volcano.

When you don't forgive, the other person is held in your energetic bondage, which will impact them negatively. But not forgiving is *far* more detrimental to the person who is holding the grudge. You are deeply hurting yourself by holding onto blame and not forgiving and releasing. Anger is toxic for the body, and consistent, vibrant health cannot be obtained if you hold onto grudges and refuse to forgive.

Forgiveness Is a Process

You may have to forgive the same person many times to clear yourself. Remember, words are powerful, and even if they don't feel true right away, the sincere desire to forgive will eventually release the stronghold of the root of resentment that is hurting your body.

I have found that you can turbocharge your forgiveness intention by calling upon the Divine within you to forgive with you and even for you. Sometimes the hurt is so deep that saying the words "I forgive you" to the other person just feels totally untrue. I encourage you to call upon your definition of the Divine to assist you: "By the power of the Divine within me, I forgive you," or perhaps more honestly, "I can't forgive you. You hurt me so much. But I want to release this anger I hold, so I am calling upon God, the Divine, the power of Love, to take away this anger and forgive for me so that I may heal myself."

Do You Also Need to Be Forgiven?

You might also realize that you are in need of forgiveness and wish to be released from someone holding onto anger and resentment toward you. The meditation for this step that I will guide you through later in this chapter will also give you an opportunity to ask for forgiveness.

We are energy beings coexisting in the quantum field. If you release judgment toward someone or ask to be released from someone else's judgment, you *are* shifting the energy. You don't have to be in direct, in-person contact with the individual to do this work. You can simply bring them into your heart by name.

In fact, there might be times when you would be wise *not* to contact someone and try to have this forgiveness conversation in person. Reconnecting with someone who traumatized you might just serve to deepen the trigger, and asking someone else for forgiveness can, in some cases, feed their painbody and sense of victimhood. So use discernment here. Let your heart guide you on this one. Start with the Forgiveness Meditation (later in this chapter) on the energetic level and see where it takes you.

You will likely have several individuals you need to forgive. As you move through the following Triggers as a Mirror exercise, you might also find that someone you didn't even know you needed to forgive arises within or that old grudges that are polluting your energy system show themselves so that you may choose to release them from your energy field.

Exercise

TRIGGERS AS A MIRROR

Before we get into our Forgiveness Meditation, let's do a brief but often revealing judgment exercise that can help loosen the ego's insistence on completely vilifying another human being.

Open your journal and think of your villain, the person you know you need to forgive and release. Now without giving it much thought, write down ten things you don't like about this person. Do it fast and be petty. You are not trying to be fair or good here. You are writing an honest list for yourself of traits that you really don't like in this other person—this person who triggers you, frankly. Ten things. Go! If you have a hard time coming up with ten, elaborate on one of the easy ones. Find a way to come up with ten. Don't read ahead until your list is complete.

Now look at your list and say before each trait, "Sometimes I am . . ." and then insert the trait. Circle the traits that are also true for you to some degree. Are those the traits that irritate you the most in the other person?

Unacknowledged shadow traits in ourselves tend to show up in others as something we don't like about them. If we see that we have some traits in common with the other person, it can make it easier for us to forgive them. We might need to include ourselves in the list of people we wish to forgive for not living up to our ideals.

JULIAN'S STORY

When my son, Julian, was eight years old, he went to my native Denmark with me for the summer. He spoke some Danish but not very much. He participated in a soccer camp near my mom's cabin, and after a game he confided, "Mama, two boys teased me because I don't speak Danish very well. But I decided to forgive one of them because his arm was in a cast. And then I decided to forgive the other one too—because it's just easier than being mad." Did Julian deserve to be mocked for his language skills? Of course not. And two against one? Come on! But he was over it. Just like that, he released it. That does make life easier, doesn't it?

Exercise

FORGIVENESS MEDITATION

Welcome to your Forgiveness Meditation. You are invited now to release the toxic vibration created by grudges, judgment, and blame.

Relax your mind by drawing your awareness to the breath. Relax your forehead and the brain behind the forehead. Allow the intellect to relax. Become more and more aware of all the little details in the breath, the sensation inside your nose as you breathe, the sensation of the breath in the back of the throat.

Feel the rise and fall of your belly and your chest. Notice the gradual slowing down of the breath as the mind starts to slow down. Bring awareness into the lower belly, below the belly button. Breathe deeply. Let the belly soften.

Feel the sensation of your breath in the back of your throat. Notice the slow rhythm of your breath and the rise and fall of your belly, your chest.

Soften the lower belly more and invite more breath in. Feel the expansion of the belly as you draw breath deep into the body. Allow the exhale to release any tension from the body and the mind. Take a deep breath in through the nose and sigh audibly out through the mouth. Feel the rhythm of your breath, and align yourself with this simple act of breathing.

Now notice your whole body in space. Notice what supports you. Notice the space around you, the sounds within you, the sounds around you.

Bring awareness to the hands. Notice the energy present in the palms of the hands, in the tips of the fingers, in the backs of the hands.

Feel your feet, and simply notice the soles of the feet, the heels, the tops of the feet, and the toes. Feel the hands and feel the feet. Feel the simple rhythmic act of breathing. Feel Spirit in the body—your Spirit Self in the body, all-loving, all-forgiving, life-giving.

Now bring awareness to the heart center. Bring your hands to the heart space, close your eyes, and ask your heart to show you who needs to be forgiven for your heart to relax. Feel the knots of unforgiveness that are constricting your heart. You know who you have to forgive to free up your heart. Whisper the name(s) to yourself: "By the power of the Divine within me, I want to forgive (name)." You might need to forgive one individual or maybe more. Maybe that one person was a stand-in for someone earlier in your life—and they, too, were a stand-in for someone even further back. If a particular kind of hurt hasn't been fully processed, it has a way of replaying itself through different people, all carrying the emotional signature of the original wound.

See what wants to happen. Close your eyes for a moment and allow the individuals who need forgiveness to rise into your awareness. Whisper the names again: "By the power of the Divine within me, I want to forgive (name)."

Now visualize each person. Let them appear behind your closed eyes. Feel the energy for a moment. Notice how your body reacts. Maybe fear and anger arise, and that's okay. You are not endorsing anything they did. You are releasing them from your judgment and blame. See this person or maybe the whole group standing before you at a safe distance. They are not here to hurt you. They are here to be released from your judgment. They are here to set you free.

Feel your loving heart. Feel the power of Infinite Spirit in your heart—Source itself. Connect deeply to your powerful heart. Now let your heart send a radiant beam of beautiful bright light directly into the hearts of the individuals standing before you. Energetically they are receiving the light from your heart. Visualize their hearts opening up to receive this light, connecting heart to heart and Spirit to Spirit. Say aloud or internally, "(Name), I forgive you. I forgive you for what you did, whether knowingly or unknowingly, through your words, thoughts, and actions, that hurt me and caused me pain." Open your heart more to this person. Let Light flow from your heart into theirs.

If it hurts, let it hurt. If you cry, let tears flow. Say again, "(Name), I forgive you. I release you from my anger. I release you from my resentment. I release you from my judgment."

Release them now from the iron grip of your anger. Let your anger soften and relax and feel your heart open more. "(Name), I forgive you. I forgive you for what you did, intentionally or unintentionally, that hurt me and caused me pain, through your thoughts, words, and actions. I forgive you now."

Allow forgiveness to fill your heart. "I forgive you. I forgive you. I forgive you." Let these words reverberate within. "By the power of the Divine within me, I forgive you, I forgive you, I forgive you." Let the Light flow from your heart, from Source itself, like a fountain of eternity, ever replenished, life itself, love itself, flowing freely now.

Now before you let these individuals go, ask yourself if you also need their forgiveness. Perhaps ask them internally. Who else might you need forgiveness from? Ask your heart. Your heart knows. Who holds resentment toward you? Who is judging and blaming you? Who carries a grudge toward you? Ask anyone you would like to ask for forgiveness to step forward.

Keep your heart open and radiating and say aloud or internally: "(Name), I ask that you forgive me now for anything and everything I did that caused you pain—anything I said, thought, or did that hurt you. I now ask that you forgive me. I am sorry. Please forgive me. Please forgive me. I am truly sorry that I hurt you."

The judging egos are not involved. This process is heart to heart, Spirit to Spirit. Feel the beam of light from your heart now, powerful and strong. Then speak these words: "By the power of the Divine within me, I now forgive everyone for anything they ever did that hurt me, intentionally or unintentionally. I release and let go of the tightness and the judgment, the anger and the hurt. I let it all go. I give it over to Divine Love. By the power of the Divine within me, I release and let go of all blame and all grudges. I release everyone from my judgment."

Continue to beam the powerful divine light from your heart into the world, then ask again for forgiveness: "Please forgive me for whatever I did to hurt you, whether I knew it or not. Please release me from your judgment. Please release any grudges and any blame you carry toward me. Please forgive me. Please release me from judgment."

Hold the steady light, thanking the individuals who received your forgiveness, and thank the individuals whose forgiveness you asked for. Thank them for appearing and thank them for what you have learned. Say to them, "May nothing be left between us except Divine Love. May nothing be left between us except Divine Love. May nothing be left between us except Divine Love." Bow your head as a sign of respect that this other person is also connected to the Divine and is also connected to Source and the Divine in you. The Divine within you and within them has now repaired the ill will, the tension, the grudges, the blame.

Let the individuals go now. Be with your heart. Feel the magnitude of the divine force of love in your heart. Feel God's presence in your heart. Feel this presence in the whole energy field of your body now. Let yourself be bathed in the powerful energy of forgiveness, bringing awareness to the whole of the body. Feel the vibration of forgiveness present in the whole of the body—in the hands and the feet, in the arms and the legs, in the torso, in all the organs, in the brain, in the face, in the hair. Feel completely enveloped in the powerful energy of forgiveness. Notice all of yourself basking in the powerful love energy of true forgiveness, which sets everyone free from the bondage of blame and judgment. Now you are free. Repeat internally or aloud: "Now I am free. Now I am free. Now I am free. God in me. God around me. God for me. God in me. God around me. God for me. God in me. God around me. God for me."

Affirmation Prayer for Forgiveness

Divine Love!

I invoke your presence within my whole being now, as I intend powerfully with all my being to forgive, release, and let go of all resentment energy that lives in my body.

I bring to mind the individuals and situations I wish to forgive, and I ask that through your powerful grace, light, and love, I now profoundly forgive and release all tight energy that would choose to hold onto resentful energy, grudges, and vindictiveness.

I let it all go by the power of your divine loving light.

If there are people and situations that I struggle to release in this manner, I now hand them over to you and allow you to release them for me so that I may now go free.

Thank you.

So be it and so it is.

Step Eight

RELATIONSHIPS AS VEHICLES FOR GROWTH

Whatever relationship you find yourself in, be it intimate or platonic, will likely serve as a mirror for you. This eighth and final step on the Heal What Hurts path is about welcoming the triggers that come up in your relationships as opportunities for continued growth as you hold yourself with loving presence.

Pause for a moment. Breathe. What has changed in the way you respond to life's triggers?

Are you able to notice the moment you are triggered? Do you feel the energetic shift in your body and your breath when someone says or does something that feels threatening to your emotional safety?

Do you notice that those around you get triggered too—and react from that place? What are the early signs that you or the other person is triggered and the two of you are heading straight into a painful dynamic that never ends well?

What does triggered energy feel like in you or in the other person? Something in the face, the eyes? The breath? Have you noticed that when you or the other person is triggered, you avoid eye contact?

When we gaze into each other's eyes for even mere seconds, we call each other back into our Spirit-guided selves. Our storytelling egos avoid that. We are in the middle of experiencing a drama that requires our spiritual essence to stay out of it, or it will collapse. Our villain projections, often accompanied by phrases like "you *always*" and "you *never*," don't stand up to the humanity of the other person. Our egos don't hold complexity well.

> *Ego-centered voice:* "You are always late and I can never trust you! You are incapable of being on time—ever!"

> *Body-centered voice:* "Sometimes you are late and it hurts and I get really scared. My solar plexus contracts and I feel small and alone. I get angry with you because the meaning I assign to it is that you don't care about me. When I feel into my body, I realize that it reminds me of the time my parents forgot to pick me up at school because they were drunk. I am embarrassed to tell you this."

> *Partner's ego-centered voice:* "I can never do anything right! You don't even care to ask what happened. I was rushing over here when a semitruck blocked the freeway and my cell phone was out of battery. I just *knew* you would get pissed and be angry, and I almost wanted to turn around and not come over!"

Partner's body-centered voice: "I am not good enough. I really wanted to be on time and I was looking forward to seeing you. But realizing how late it was, I was scared to walk into your house. I knew you would be disappointed in me. I hate disappointing you. It reminds me of my dad and how I always missed the mark. When you lecture me, I feel like a fifth grader and I lose my capacity to think straight in the face of your anger. I just want to run away and hide."

Next time you and your partner are triggered, can you pause, breathe, and be centered in yourself?

Gaze into each other's eyes. Maybe even smile.

Then communicate from the felt sensation in the body:

- "My body is feeling tense. How is your body?"
- "My breathing does not feel free and open. Does yours?"
- "My heart is beating a little faster. Can we pause, please?"
- "Can we help each other inquire into what is happening between us?"
- "Can we identify what stories we are each experiencing right now?"
- "Can we just be quiet and gaze into each other's eyes for a full minute? Can we smile while we do it, even if it feels forced?"

If the two of you are able to slow things down and stay grounded in your bodies, there is hope that you will communicate something much truer and more vulnerable to your partner—something that may be triggered by their action, yes, but is reinforced and magnified by a matching trigger. Having cultivated increased awareness of the energy field of your body, you are no longer quite so likely to go on autopilot and react according to an old story that may or may not be replaying in the present. Or at least you might be able to recognize that you are triggered and that there are two stories happening at the same time and they need to be separated.

There are the objective facts and then there is the story that each of you create about them—your interpretation of the facts: "You are late and it triggers a time when my parents being late really did mean that they had more important priorities than being my parents. Your being late today may not mean that I am not important to you. If I can slow down and realize that I am merging these stories, then I can avoid interpreting my partner's lateness with something far more traumatic, like parents forgetting a child. Then I can get an objective sense of what is going on." It is indeed possible that you really are not important to your partner, but if the old story is playing simultaneously, you can't see clearly.

You may or may not have a partner who is conscious enough or interested enough in doing this trigger healing work with you, but *you* can realize that an old script has been unleashed, whether it's within you or your partner—or both simultaneously, as is so often the case. That means you can guide the divine presence within you to swoop in and truly hold that terrified part of you that is reliving a scary experience of not feeling loved, safe, or like you belong.

Conscious Partners Can Coevolve Through a Trigger

If you can slow down enough to share the resurfacing of old pain with your partner, then your partner might even assist you in becoming present with yourself. The opposite might also be true: You see your partner go into a triggered state and you are able to help them feel into the body and locate a contracted place within that needs presence. *That is a coevolving relationship.* It will hurt at times, because you have both picked a partner who has an uncanny ability to activate your triggers, but through your dedicated practice of the steps in this book, you will have enough present moment awareness to stop, breathe, feel your body, and not allow your respective scripts to run off with you. That will not always work, but it must mostly work if you are to create a safe union with each other, and then the soul growth potential is limitless.

From a yogic perspective, triggers may well have accumulated for lifetimes and it is not realistic to think that either of you will ever be trigger-free. The key to a *coevolving relationship* is that each partner takes responsibility for their state of mind and for the story that the trigger releases when activated. It ultimately requires that each of you commit to at least mostly giving up any of the three common trigger reactions: lashing out, numbing out, and checking out. That is easier said than done, but it can help tremendously if you get really clear on your go-to *outs* and very honest about when you are headed for one of them.

If you insist on resorting to any of the three trigger reactions, you are cutting yourself off from the light of the Divine that is needed for true healing. Eventually you will realize that the relationship is a dead end and will not lead to growth or a deepening of love but instead will harm you both—and leave both of you with tighter trigger knots.

When you approach the fine and difficult art of mastering your triggers and choose to stay present in the body, allowing yourself to be vulnerable and honest instead of reactive, you will begin to see your partner realistically. You have in effect taken off your trigger-tinted, blurred, or even completely distorted glasses. You are now looking objectively at your partner's behavior and habits. Your body is no longer flooding you with stress when they do that thing, but you may still realize that a given behavior is so entrenched in your partner and simply doesn't line up with your values.

That is very different from going into reaction. You are no longer a child reacting to a perceived threat; you are an adult calmly observing another person's choices in the world, and you are now making wise and mature decisions for yourself and even for your partner.

If you leave your partner on a trigger-reactive note, chances are the very same trigger will draw to you a similar situation that will once more invite you to come into presence with the contracted trigger knot so that you may love it into wholeness.

Remember, the trigger knot is like a speck on your projected Light and can't *not* show up in your life again. If, on the other hand, you have held yourself, your fear, your contracted energy, in sincere self-love, then you are free. Because now you can look at the people around you and assess very calmly whether their vibration is one that you choose to have in your intimate sphere.

Your Inner Vibration Becomes Your Lived Experience

As you change your vibration into one of presence and self-love, anyone who is not truly treating you with love and kindness will likely cease to be of interest to you, and you to them. The vibrational match is simply not there anymore.

Changing your relationship is an inside job. What is present on the inside will manifest on the outside. Your mind is not the best tool to ascertain whether a partner is right for you. You will ultimately feel it in your body. Do you mostly feel safe and chosen with your partner? Are the two of you creating a strong container in which the triggers that are inevitable in an intimate relationship can be processed?

Your Relationship Will Always Be a Sacred Mirror

Any relationship you find yourself in, whether intimate or platonic, will likely serve as a mirror for you. Whatever triggers you have will show you where you need more loving presence. When the triggering gift of a given relationship has revealed itself fully and you no longer look to your partner to fill a need that you were previously not willing to fill for yourself, you have set yourself free to choose wisely. The dramatic feelings have subsided and you are in effect a true adult making a wise partner choice for yourself. Now you are free to look at the other person with some degree of detachment and can ask yourself:

- Do we have enough common ground here to build a life together?
- Do we have a similar code of conduct?
- Are we relatively clear on our own and the other person's triggers?
- Can we each take full responsibility for our wounds while being willing to empathically hold the other in their ongoing healing?
- Are we in agreement about what level of commitment we want?
- What are our shared values? Where do we differ?
- What is our shared agreement in regard to the amount of time spent together, plans made together, and the degree to which we each wish to pursue separate goals, adventures, and relationships?
- What is my biggest challenge in terms of the other person's personality? Can I live with it? Truly?
- What degree of commitment am I hoping for (financial, practical, professional, housing, family, friends)?
- Do I want to be legally married or have a spiritual commitment ceremony? Why or why not?

- If we are of childbearing age, do we want kids? How will we share in raising kid(s)?

The list can go on and on, but it won't be that hard to make once it's no longer being compiled by two kids fighting to be loved and recognized but rather two adults fully willing to be present for themselves and for each other—willing to own their own triggers, trace the origin of the triggers in the energy field of the body, and have the ongoing courage to hold themselves when triggered.

When you both get skilled at staying and loving and being present with yourself (and even with each other) when the trigger process has been set in motion, you are approaching emotional liberation. Yet chances are you will slip up every now and then. In fact, in my coaching practice I have not met anyone (and certainly not myself) who gets this on the first, second, or even third try. Triggers can be dense and tough, and the way they start to heal is by *not* acting out of them but instead holding them, feeling them, and being present with them and not allowing the story that is being released to drive the bus.

The situation that has triggered you for a lifetime will likely still give you butterflies, and if the trigger is still locked away, it will find a way to draw in the kind of person who will poke at it. Even after you have loved it and held it, it may still erupt, but gradually to a lesser degree. And you will slowly but surely cultivate more space within yourself to pause and breathe and hold it in love.

You Will Still Get Triggered, and That's Normal

Don't be disappointed if you still slip into at least a mini version of what used to become a full-blown drama. The deepest triggers haven't necessarily disappeared, but you have learned to hold them in a different way.

If you consider your trigger knot to be a speck in your *citta* (your heart-mind energy field, or what we might simply call the energy field of the body) being projected out into your life experience, then you will realize that whoever and whatever surrounds you is a pretty accurate indication of what lies within.

The Ongoing Work of Healing Your Triggers

Let's talk about how you can continue the work of healing your triggers going forward. While this process has been laid out for you in a step-by-step fashion, the truth is it's an ongoing and circular process. You will need breath and body awareness forever and you will need to cultivate ever more consistent unconditional love for yourself forever. Those are your primary tools in this work.

I recommend that you set some positive intentions for how you do this work, especially with other people, because that is where this work becomes apparent. If we lived in a vacuum, we wouldn't meet these places within ourselves. It is predominantly in relationships that our deepest triggers flare up. Because you now have a good sense of how you breathe and you have a good sense of the energy system of your body, you will know very early on, "Oh, I'm triggered! Something is going on here that

I need to look at. I'm going to take space. I'm going to inquire inwardly. I'm going to find out what my story is here, and the story will not run off with my nervous system and reactions as it has probably done for years, maybe even decades."

How Do I Know If a Relationship Is Worth Working On?

Obviously there are relationships that are truly unhealthy, where two people continually trigger each other at the deepest level, with no awareness of their own part in the drama. The less conscious we are and the deeper the triggers, the more likely we are to be caught in a vicious cycle of emotional reactivity and compulsive behavior.

Nevertheless, the relationship shows us something about ourselves. It always takes two to tango. If one person gets triggered and the other stays truly calm and present, the triggered dynamic loses momentum. One person may appear calm but in reality be checked out, while the other person appears to be in extreme reaction. That is still a trigger dynamic. When we look at emotionally reactive dynamics through the lens of the three *outs*, we often see one person defaulting to lashing out while the other tends to check out. These patterns reinforce each other: The more one person lashes out, the more the other withdraws, and the more that person checks out, the more agitated and reactive the other becomes. It's a painful cycle, where each person's coping mechanism exacerbates the other's.

Numbing out can also enter the equation—sometimes used by both people to avoid discomfort altogether. But the numbing agent itself (such as alcohol, scrolling, or food) often magnifies the primary reaction. A person prone to lashing out may become more volatile when numbing—think of having a drink and firing off a barrage of late-night texts. A person prone to checking out may become even more distant—having a drink and disappearing emotionally for the rest of the night. Instead of diffusing tension, numbing tends to intensify the very behaviors we're trying to escape.

If you find yourself in this painful dynamic, just know that either behavior will exacerbate it. Both people are hurting in this scenario, and taking space is likely the only way to release from the gridlock.

At some point you might have to look at a relationship and decide if it is a coevolving relationship where each person is able to learn and grow from the encounter and ultimately take the relationship to higher ground. Take a close look at where the two of you are with your *outs*. If you have mostly given up your *outs*, it may not be productive or supportive for you to partner with someone who is still mostly resorting to an *out*. You will likely not be an energetic match for each other anymore.

Going in makes you ever more present, and you will begin to require that same level of presence from your partner. Presence is like the wattage of a light bulb: Turning inward increases the wattage, while resorting to an *out* dims it. If you are working diligently with the Heal What Hurts method, it's very likely that you have become a higher-wattage light bulb—and you will naturally attract and be attracted to someone of a similar caliber. The more present you are, the more love you exude. You will want to be met by someone who is your equal.

Whoever meets you in your close relationships is a mirror image of what lies within. The best bet for finding a high-caliber partner is to do your own inner work—not with the goal of finding a partner, but with the purpose of becoming the highest, most illuminated version of yourself and bringing your light to the world. If you get lost in the *outs* with your partner, the world is missing out on your presence.

If a relationship seems to do little more than play out in painful ways over and over, with the individuals unable to self-reflect and take responsibility, then the triggers are likely being driven deeper and deeper into the energy field of the body. You can leave such a painful scenario, but if you don't explore the inner reasons for your part in the dynamic, it is very likely that you will play out a similar drama with someone else.

The physiological impact of being in a triggered state is one of stress, pure and simple. If you could measure your heart rate and the level of cortisol and adrenaline in your blood when you are going into a state of being triggered, you would see very clearly that you are in physical as much as emotional distress.

Rob, a trauma nurse who participated in my online Heal What Hurts program, shared an experience where he had a patient hooked up to a monitor, which made her vitals visible in numbers. She was in great emotional distress, making her veins collapse. Having learned about his own triggers, Rob knew that calming the patient down naturally was possible if she could be in her body and slow her breathing. So he quietly guided her to calm and deepen her breath while feeling systematically into her body. Within minutes her vitals stabilized and her veins regained their healthy volume, avoiding further intervention.

The purpose of the meditation for this step is to set a positive note for what we want in our relationship. What kind of relationships do we want so that we can continue to grow and can contribute to somebody else's growth? We also open ourselves to the possibility that a given relationship might have to fall away if it's not for our highest mutual growth. Can you each take full responsibility for your triggers?

I have not met very many people willing to go so deeply in and take complete responsibility for their own life experience. It is the ultimate act of love to hold the places that really hurt but also understand that the story was born out of that hurt and has played out enough, and now it's time for it to stop. When that story is no longer playing out, you can allow a new, beautiful story of your life to unfold. Your creative Spirit can flow through this beautiful vessel of your body that has become a much healthier instrument, with fewer knots.

I can't wait to hear from you about how you experience the wholeness of this process and what's unfolding in your life. You're welcome to share your reflections with me via my website: www.mariatoso.com. There's always more room for growth. There's always more creative power that we can give birth to.

Exercise

COEVOLVING RELATIONSHIP MEDITATION

Welcome to your Coevolving Relationship Meditation.

Begin by centering yourself, by being fully present in your body. Notice your breath. Calmly inhale all the way into the lower belly. Let the whole body relax as you exhale and let go.

Inhale to fill up all the way as the lower belly expands. Let go and relax—and notice where your body feels open and at ease and where there might be tightness, holding, or contraction. Where does something feel off? Just observe, without judgment. Your body is your sacred road map, and your intuition and knowing will speak to you through the energy field of the body.

Over the past eight weeks you have become very capable of noticing the subtle energetic vibrations of the body. You have grown in your ability to be present in the whole energy field of the body and not get lost so much in the thought world of the mind.

This meditation is your invitation to check in with the relationships you have. Is the company you keep for your highest growth, or is it to your detriment? Let your body give you the answers you seek.

Let yourself truly feel into the body, starting at the top of the head. Feel the scalp, the ears, and the forehead. Feel into the little muscles around the eyes and the nose. Notice the cool stream of air inside the nose. Notice your lips, your tongue, your teeth. Notice your chin and your throat. Feel into the muscles in the back of the neck, the sides of your neck. Let any tension melt away from the shoulders.

Notice the shoulder blades and the muscles around the shoulder blades. Release and relax. Notice the right side of the chest and the left side, from the collarbones to the breastbone. Feel the belly and the side ribs. Feel your lower back. Notice your hips, your thighs and knees, your lower legs and ankles. Notice the heels and the soles of your feet and the tops of the feet.

Notice your toes. Feel the shoulders and upper arms and elbows. Feel the wrists, the hands, the fingers. Feel the palms of the hands, the backs of the hands, the fingertips. Fully embody yourself. Notice everything that's going on within, objectively observing, feeling, noticing, breathing.

Now invite your body to communicate with you. How do the energy fields of other individuals impact you? Sometimes individuals provoke triggers so that we may see them, but they are truly innocent in doing so.

Other times triggers are there to show us where these injuries are, and when we have truly owned them within us, the individual who triggered these places may no longer have a place in our life.

Bring to mind an individual in your life who is a close ally but you're questioning whether it should stay that way. Continue to stay very grounded in your body. As you bring this individual closer to mind, be very observant of any energetic vibrational messages in your body.

As this individual comes closer to mind at your invitation, what is the vibration between the two of you? Does this person support your growth? What is the quality of the connection between the two of you? Is it truly love, or is it something else—like attachment, longing, or projection? Real love feels different. It's not about needing the other person to complete us; it's about how deeply we want to show up for them. When we truly love someone, we want to say to them: "I'm here. I love you. I've got you." We long to meet each other in realness, beyond the roles and facades, and to be known in our vulnerability as well as our strength.

But here's the heart of it: We cannot truly offer that kind of love to another until we've learned to offer it to ourselves. The very words we are learning to speak inwardly—"I'm here, I love you, I've got you"—we long to extend outward when our own cup is full. Without self-love, what we call "love" often turns into a draining string of self-sacrifice. But when love flows from the inner well that is always being filled by the Divine within, it doesn't feel like sacrifice—it feels like overflow.

Feel the energy field of the body. Steer clear of the intellect, which may try to interject stories. You're asking the Spirit that lives in the body. Do you want this individual to come closer? Is there warmth? Is there kindness? Does this individual feed you on some level with their energy? Is there a nurturing quality? A caring quality? What is the quality of this individual? Does the energy feel expansive or contracted?

Where do you feel the presence of this individual in your body now? There may be more than one area of the energy field of the body acting up. Choose the loudest one right now and bring your awareness to that place.

You may lay your hand on this place in the body. How does it feel to have this individual in your life? You don't have to draw a conclusion—it doesn't have to be a clear yes or no. Just notice all the information available.

Are you loved by this individual? Do you love this individual? Do you feel safe with this individual? Is there compassion between the two of you? Sexual love is the seed and compassion is the flower. Do you feel that this person wants to support you, lift you up, and enhance your life? Is that what you want to do for this person? Do you see each other's vulnerability and tenderness and do you feel held by each other?

Is this a person you would leave a small child or your favorite pet with for the day? Is this the person you would call at 2:00 a.m. if you were in trouble? Could they call you? Are you there for each other? Can you genuinely say to each other, "I love you, I am here, I've got you"? In this book you have learned to say that to yourself. For a relationship to be viable, you both must feel that your own love cup overflows to the point that you can include another in that level of love. Are you there? Can you imagine growing into that with this person? Is your sexual chemistry loving and good? Do you feel safe in this person's arms and vice versa?

Do you belong in each other's lives? What does your body say? What are the feelings that arise? Can you put words to any feelings that arise within the body?

Now invite this individual to come closer. What happens in your body? Be honest. Observe all the vibrations in your body now.

Now invite this individual to step farther away, much farther away. What happens in your body?

Now invite this individual to step completely out of your energy field. Stay in touch with the vibrations that remain in your body after this visit from this individual.

Does this individual belong in your life? Does this individual have a sacred place in your life? Is it time to say goodbye to this individual?

When you say or think of the word *goodbye* in regard to this individual, what feelings arise? If you think the words *stay, be in my life*, what feelings and vibrations are in the body?

Now release all the words. Put your hands on your heart and ask inwardly, "What do I need to know in regard to this person?" What arises? Words? Feelings? Scenarios?

Release your hands from your heart as you thank your heart for communicating with you.

Promise yourself to continue to check in at this level—not through the intellect, not through analyzing, but at this deeply energetic level, where the body gets to communicate and be heard.

In this final step on the Heal What Hurts path, the body is no longer an afterthought. By now, you are walking in a different body—one that is more awake, more felt, more trusted. Through each step you've learned to soften into sensation, stay present with discomfort, and listen rather than override. You numb less. You abandon yourself less. The body is now honored as a wise, living instrument—vibrantly alive and always in conversation with the energy within and around you. You move through the world with a deeper sense of inner contact because the body is no longer a battlefield or a burden—it's home.

Silently make the following promise to your beautiful, radiant body that is the sacred road map of your journey: "I will pay attention. I will be very deeply present in my body. I will not numb out the messages from my body. I will listen. I will check in. I want this information. Thank you for being willing to communicate with me. I am here. I love you."

Slowly open your eyes. Look around the space where you are. See what's there. Feel the vibrancy and aliveness of the body that is loved and respected and honored by you.

Walk in this world with this body that is full of love, in which you are fully present and fully loving, surrounded by love, inviting in love, ever raising your vibration. Feel into the vibrant, creative, brilliant soul that you are: potent with your unique soul mission to be carried out by you in this world, walking in love, knowing that you are safe and that you belong, walking with Divine Love inside you always.

Affirmation Prayer for Relationships

Divine Love!

I call upon your loving light-filled presence to imbue any and all of my relationships with your awareness, that I may see clearly, through your wisdom and grace, whether a relationship is for the highest good of both individuals, for growing ever closer to our own divinity by shedding layer upon layer of old pain that we have projected on each other.

That your loving light will make it clear when and if a relationship has served its purpose or still has more to teach each of us about loving one another and ourselves with the compassion and grace that is the Divine within.

Thank you.

So be it and so it is.

A WHOLE NEW PARADIGM FOR FRIENDSHIP

Much of human communication is the sharing of stories and beliefs and how those stories and beliefs show up in—or downright shape—our relationships. We tend to paint ourselves as the victim of a given situation and then recruit support for that view. It feels good to have someone else agree with how we view things. We tend to think of a good friend as someone who can see *our* side of things and make us feel validated in our story. Often our story about not being treated right reminds the other person of all the ways *they* have not been treated right—and together we can agree that *we* are good people and some other person or group is lacking in goodness.

Painbodies Egging Each Other On

The problem is that essentially our wounded self, or painbody, is being encouraged by other painbodies to spiral further downward in our trigger stories. And while we *do* need empathy, support, and understanding, we need that energy to be applied to the contracted energy in the body—not to strengthen the *story* and beliefs held in that knot.

Let me explain. Let's return to the story I told at the beginning of the book of how my husband didn't call me before bedtime when he was out of town and I felt a tremendous contracted trigger pain inside. In this situation, I could have called a friend of mine and told her my trigger knot story: *He is a jerk. He doesn't love me. I should probably get divorced. He is just not up for conscious partnership. He might be having an affair.*

And if, at that point, my friend had enthusiastically agreed with some version of my story—"I agree, all of this is very likely. He is indeed very bad. It's not the first time you have dealt with this. You have to do something. Maybe it's time to leave"—then with her words she would have poured gasoline on my story, which was already on fire, and my lashing out would have been amplified.

Or, on the flip side, she could have said, "You are freaking out. Stop crying. You don't know if any of this is true. You are so dramatic. Why don't you just go to sleep? Take a chill pill." She could have shamed me for freaking out and essentially encouraged me to find another *out*: "Go ahead, numb out, check out."

Instead, my friend could say to me, "I am here. I am sorry you are hurting. I love you. I am not going anywhere. I am right here. Are you willing to breathe deeply and connect with your body? I will be right here with you as you feel your body. Where do you feel contracted, Maria?"

At that point, I might slow down my storytelling, close my eyes, breathe consciously, and become aware that my heart center is contracted: "I can barely breathe. I will relax as best I can and breathe deeply. I feel the fear of losing my husband mixed in with the pain of having lost my dad." Then I cry and the story subsides. Now I am just with the felt sense in my body. It becomes a lump in my throat. I describe these sensations to my friend. She says, "I am here, Maria. I am here with you." Slowly my heart starts to relax and my breathing becomes calmer. I no longer feel like spewing. I am just quietly aware of old pain dissipating from my heart center. My friend stays on the phone with me until I feel done. The cloud has lifted.

That's a different way of being a friend. She never even gives me a sense of whether she thinks I should get divorced or take a chill pill, because she doesn't know. She just knows I am in distress and it is easier for me to be present with my pain when she is right there lending me her presence, her love, and her compassion as I enter my pained, contracted heart and allow myself to really feel it and release. My heart is softer now. I can sleep now.

Ideally we would also be a good new-paradigm friend to our romantic partner. This, of course, can happen only if one partner stays at least relatively untriggered and the triggered partner has not descended too far into one of their *outs*. The recognition that a trigger has been activated has to be almost immediate. In my experience, if we don't catch it quickly, we tend to default to one of our habitual *outs*. But the body always signals the shift right away. With deep awareness of what's happening in your body and breath, you can learn to recognize a trigger as it arises and choose to go inward instead of acting out. From there, both partners need to realize that triggered energy can be traced in the body. If the triggering issue is one that involves both of you, it will be harder to resolve but it can be achieved.

Triggers Often Mirror Each Other

James and Marianne did a heroic job working on the triggers that arose in their relationship. One night Marianne got triggered when James announced that he had made plans without her for the next day. Her typical *out* was to lash out and let James know what she thought about that, but in this case she used all her inner tools to contain the urge. Instead, she got quiet as she continued cooking—but simultaneously she worked on calling on Divine Love to help her be present for the contracted energy in her body and to fill her heart with radiant love. She could feel the story well up: *He doesn't prioritize me. Something else is more important or someone else is more important.* It tied right back to feelings she had with her dad, who had traveled during most of her childhood.

James sensed her falling quiet and was prodding her: "Why are you quiet? What's going on?"

Marianne let him know that she was just processing some energy in her body that needed her presence. And lo and behold, her silence triggered James and he burst out, "So now you're keeping secrets? Now you're not letting me know what's going on with you!"

In that moment, Marianne was able to say to James, "I am here. Can we work through this? Can we sit and look each other in the eye for a moment and feel what's going on here?"

James agreed. It's not important who was able to ask the question, but in this case it was Marianne: "James, I love you and I am here. Are you willing to feel your body right now?"

James agreed, closed his eyes, deepened his shallow breathing, and scanned his torso. His hand reached to his heart and his chin quivered. "I am right here," said Marianne as she imagined a beam of Divine Love radiating from her heart into his while she empathically held his hand.

Then James spoke: "I have a memory of being sixteen years old. I am at an outfitters store in Montana with my dad. It is supposed to be our time together, camping and fly fishing, but he is constantly on the phone in the corner of the store. Every time I edge near him, he says loudly into the phone, "Oh, now James is right here next to me."

Somehow James knew that his dad was on the phone with his secretary, who had become a lot more than a secretary. "He was keeping secrets from me," said James. "I felt shut out. Even though we had driven all the way to Montana together, my dad wasn't present with me at all." James wept a bit, and the two of them hugged.

Curiously, the trigger had started with Marianne feeling shut out, then James felt shut out, and through loving presence they were both able to feel into the body how their fathers had felt absent and how much it had hurt to feel shut out by them.

This is a beautiful example of a couple who was able to take what started out as relatively minor bickering and turn it into an opportunity to heal something that stemmed back to each of their childhoods. It must be said that this couple had a lot of practice and plenty of examples of not being able to find each other in the heat of a trigger.

Realistically, it's always going to be easier to do this process with a friend in a situation where you have no stake in the game. If whatever is triggering them is not because of something you did, that will make it easier for you to simply hold space for them to feel their body and call upon Divine Love and to reassure them of your presence and love. The key is to stop and feel your body, whether you are alone, with a friend, or with a partner. Developing that degree of awareness can take time, especially if there have been a lot of numbing agents involved in the *out* of one or both partners. Doing the breath and body awareness meditations is key.

What to Remember If You Are Holding Space for Another

When you hold space for someone, be as present as you can in your own body. Notice every sensation that arises. Ask the person if they are willing to simply feel their body and breathe, and reassure them of your intention to hold loving presence for them: "I am here. I want to be here for you." If they are defensive with you or too far gone in their triggered state, it likely will not work. It's okay. Just back off. The opening is not there for you to hold space for them. Maybe some other time.

If they say yes, then guide them to feel their body. Send them loving compassion. Let them know, "I am here. I love you. I am not going anywhere. I just want to sit here with you." Give space, silence, presence. Imagine a beam of light radiating Divine Love from your heart to theirs. If they start up with a story about what they remember, listen, but if you hear them stray from the felt sensation and the pure memory, gently guide them back to the body. Keep reminding them to breathe and feel their body. Keep sending them Divine Love from your heart to theirs. Just be there. Many people don't really trust that anyone would want to just be there and hold space for them and love them and not be in a hurry to move on to the next thing. "I am here. There is nowhere I would rather be than here with you. Take as long as it takes. I've got you."

When we bicker, a lot of words fly through the ether—from us, to us—and rarely do any of these words cast light on anything, soothe anyone, or explain anything. They are just mindless, careless words darting back and forth. There are two contracted egos desperately trying to impose their version of reality on each other. It doesn't work. Let's be real. *It does not work.* Withdraw, pull out, give up. You are not going to get what you need from that dynamic. If you are not able to go into your bodies together, you have to do it separately.

If, on the other hand, you both sincerely want to create a Heal What Hurts union with a partner, the only way is *in*, going in together, making it your business to become radiantly present in your body.

APPROACHING YOUR LIFE WITH YOUR NEW TOOLS

For the longest time I believed that a trigger-free life was the goal of my spiritual practice. *Then* I would finally be happy and carefree, get my happily ever after, if you will—and not have to experience the pain within. I don't believe that anymore. I don't even want that anymore.

Wanting to be free of being triggered is akin to loving life and myself conditionally—as in, I can do this life thing and be there for myself only if I don't have to hold myself through pain. That's not what I am here for anymore. I am here to experience the unconditional love within me, the Divine Love within me, toward myself and from there toward the world, life, and all the other struggling souls.

When I experience being triggered about life, when I'm feeling insecure about being safe and loved and belonging, I now abandon myself less with the *outs*: lashing out, numbing out, or checking out. I am now more likely to rush in to *be with me* in deep, deep presence inside, holding my beloved self in all my anguish. I speak words of reassurance to myself, the very words I missed hearing when I was little and scared and felt powerless:

"I am here. I've got you. I know you feel shame and fear and, more than anything, sadness. I understand and I am here to hold you while you allow those feelings to surface and release. If you need to cry, I am here. If you need to walk in the woods, I am here. I am with you and I love you. You cannot lose my love, even if you act out and lash out, numb out, or check out. I will be right here waiting to hold you as you process the shame of reacting and let yourself sink into my arms of love and you finally understand that I love you now and always."

LIVING THE HEAL WHAT HURTS WAY

If you have truly practiced the steps on the Heal What Hurts path, you have most likely realized that your emotional triggers are not enemies to be suppressed or problems to be fixed, but are sacred invitations. Each one points to a place in your energy field, your body, your past, where love has not yet fully arrived—and by the power of your loving presence you lead divinity straight into those places to transform the contracted pain into love.

This path is not a one-time fix. This is a new way of living—living in love for yourself, for your body.

To live the Heal What Hurts way is to become raw and honest and endlessly compassionate with yourself; to walk with God—not as an abstract belief, but as a living presence that meets you from within every time you choose to stay, to soften, and to love and hold what hurts.

You may still get triggered.

You may still forget and lash out, numb out, or check out.

But now you know how to come back.

You know how to pause.

To breathe.

To listen.

To enter the body.

To find the contracted place.

To ask what it remembers.

To stay with it in love until it softens or reveals something true.

You know how to hold what hurts with presence until it softens.

You are no longer living from the wound. You are living from wholeness.

When you do this—day by day, moment by moment—you begin to walk with more peace. You stop grasping outside yourself for safety, for validation, for love itself. You know where it lives now: within.

And you become, slowly but surely, a transmission of that love into the world. The more you hold yourself in loving presence, the more you become that presence—not as a performance, but as a lived frequency, an inner broadcast of wholeness that others can feel.

You don't need to force anything anymore. You are aligned. You are becoming who you were always meant to be.

Affirmation Prayer for the Heal What Hurts Path

Beloved divine presence, thank you for guiding me through the healing of what hurts.

I affirm now that I am ready to live differently. I no longer abandon myself in fear or reaction. I choose to stay. To soften. To witness. To love.

When a trigger arises, I will remember: This is not an attack. It is a doorway.

I will meet what hurts with tenderness. I will listen to the voice within me that was never heard. I will comfort the places in me that were never held. I will breathe with the child in me that was never protected.

I remember now that love is not something I must earn or chase. Love is what I am made of. Love is my native language. Love is my true vibration.

I walk with God now—not outside of me, but within me. The Divine lives in my breath, in my body, in my being. The Divine lives in my heart.

I am willing to be present. I am willing to do the inner work. And through that sacred willingness, I change the world around me.

I place a different vibration into the world—one of presence, of compassion, of peace. I stand in compassionate presence within myself, fully embodied, fully alive.

I am no longer ruled by the past. I am no longer frozen in pain.

I am no longer waiting for permission to feel whole.

I am already whole. I am already free. I am already enough.

I bless my path. I bless my body. I bless my heart. I bless this day. I bless my life.

I am walking in the Heal What Hurts way. And I will never walk alone.

So be it. And so it is.

ACKNOWLEDGMENTS AND GRATITUDE

This book would not have seen the light of day had I not connected with Suzanne O'Brien and Lori Hughes, talented editors who helped me see that this book was important to get out to more people and helped me find my fabulous editors at Llewellyn, Liz Stewart and Andrea Neff. I call you my book's midwives.

And let's be real: Had it not been for my romantic partners in life, I would not have been made aware of the deep trigger knots that I carry in my body. Each in your own way has helped me find the path to heal my emotional triggers.

To Write to the Author

If you wish to contact the author or would like more information about this book, please write to the author in care of Llewellyn Worldwide Ltd. and we will forward your request. Both the author and the publisher appreciate hearing from you and learning of your enjoyment of this book and how it has helped you. Llewellyn Worldwide Ltd. cannot guarantee that every letter written to the author can be answered, but all will be forwarded. Please write to:

Maria Toso
℅ Llewellyn Worldwide
2143 Wooddale Drive
Woodbury, MN 55125-2989

Please enclose a self-addressed stamped envelope for reply, or $1.00 to cover costs. If outside the U.S.A., enclose an international postal reply coupon.

Many of Llewellyn's authors have websites with additional information and resources. For more information, please visit our website at http://www.llewellyn.com.